LEAN AND GREEN DIET COOKBOOK:

The Ultimate Complete Guide on How to Rapidly Lose Weight Following Lean and Green Diet Plan Without Stress. A 28-Days Meal Plan and Shopping List for Each Week

LEAN AND GREEN DIET COOKBOOK:

© Copyright 2020 - All rights reserved.

The content contained within this book may not be reproduced, duplicated or transmitted without direct written permission from the author or the publisher. Under no circumstances will any blame or legal responsibility be held against the publisher, or author, for any damages, reparation, or monetary loss due to the information contained within this book. Either directly or indirectly.

Legal Notice:

This book is copyright protected. This book is only for personal use. You cannot amend, distribute, sell, use, quote or paraphrase any part, or the content within this book, without the consent of the author or publisher.

Disclaimer Notice:

Please note the information contained within this document is for educational and entertainment purposes only. All effort has been executed to present accurate, up to date, and reliable, complete information. No warranties of any kind are declared or implied. Readers acknowledge that the author is not engaging in the rendering of legal, financial, medical or professional advice. The content within this book has been derived from various sources. Please consult a licensed professional before attempting any techniques outlined in this book.

By reading this document, the reader agrees that under no circumstances is the author responsible for any losses, direct or indirect, which are incurred as a result of the use of information contained within this document, including, but not limited to, errors, omissions, or inaccuracies.

LEAN AND GREEN DIET COOKBOOK:

Table of Contents

INTRODUCTION 8
    HOW TO START THIS DIET? 8
    HOW TO FOLLOW THE LEAN AND GREEN DIET? 9
    THE BENEFITS OF LEAN AND GREEN DIET 10

CHAPTER 1: FUNDAMENTALS OF LEAN AND GREEN PROGRAM 12
    5&1 LEAN AND GREEN DIET PLAN 13
    4&2&1 LEAN AND GREEN DIET PLAN 13
    3&3 LEAN AND GREEN DIET PLAN 13

CHAPTER 2: HOW DOES LEAN AND GREEN WORK? 14

CHAPTER 3: RECOMMENDED FOOD THAT ARE ALLOWED AND NOT ALLOWED 16
    FOODS THAT ARE ALLOWED 16
    FOODS THAT ARE NOT ALLOWED 19

CHAPTER 4: LEAN AND GREEN RECIPES 20
1. ADOBO SIRLOIN 20
2. BEEF STROGANOFF 21
3. SAVORY BURGERS 22
4. BEEF LO MEIN 22
5. BEEF LASAGNA 23
6. TERIYAKI SIRLOIN STEAKS 24
7. SALISBURY STEAK 25
8. BEEF AND CHICKEN SAUSAGE-STUFFED MINI PEPPERS 26
9. GRILLED ROSEMARY LAMB CHOPS 27
10. HONEY-MUSTARD LEG OF LAMB 28
11. PORK CHOPS BRAISED WITH ORANGES 28
12. PLUM SAUCE-GLAZED PORK CHOPS 29
13. DIJON AND SAGE-COATED PORK TENDERLOIN 30
14. SMOTHERED CAJUN PORK CHOPS WITH TOMATOES 30
15. PESTO ZUCCHINI NOODLES 31
16. BAKED COD & VEGETABLES 32
17. PARMESAN ZUCCHINI 33
18. CHICKEN ZUCCHINI NOODLES 33
19. TOMATO CUCUMBER AVOCADO SALAD 34
20. CREAMY CAULIFLOWER SOUP 35
21. TACO ZUCCHINI BOATS 36
22. BROCCOLI SALAD 37
23. ZUCCHINI QUICHE 37
24. TURKEY SPINACH EGG MUFFINS 38
25. CHICKEN CASSEROLE 39
26. ALOO GOBI 40
27. JACKFRUIT CARNITAS 40
28. BAKED BEANS 41
29. BRUSSELS SPROUTS CURRY 42
30. JAMBALAYA 43
31. MUSHROOM-KALE STROGANOFF 44
32. TOMATILLO AND GREEN CHILI PORK STEW ... 44
33. AVOCADO LIME SHRIMP SALAD 45
34. GRILLED MAHI-MAHI WITH JICAMA SLAW ... 46
35. ROSEMARY CAULIFLOWER ROLLS 47

CHAPTER 5: BREAKFAST 48
36. ALKALINE BLUEBERRY SPELT PANCAKES 48
37. ALKALINE BLUEBERRY MUFFINS 49
38. CRUNCHY QUINOA MEAL 49
39. COCONUT PANCAKES 50
40. QUINOA PORRIDGE 51
41. AMARANTH PORRIDGE 51
42. BANANA BARLEY PORRIDGE 52
43. ZUCCHINI MUFFINS 53
44. MILLET PORRIDGE 53
45. JACKFRUIT VEGETABLE FRY 54
46. ZUCCHINI PANCAKES 55
47. SQUASH HASH 55
48. HEMP SEED PORRIDGE 56
49. PUMPKIN SPICE QUINOA 56
50. CHOCOLATE CHERRY CRUNCH GRANOLA 57
51. MANGO COCONUT OATMEAL 58
52. SCRAMBLED EGGS WITH SOY SAUCE AND BROCCOLI SLAW 59
53. TASTY BREAKFAST DONUTS 60
54. CHEESY SPICY BACON BOWLS 60
55. GOAT CHEESE ZUCCHINI KALE QUICHE 61
56. RICOTTA RAMEKINS 62
57. CHICKEN LO MEIN 63
58. PANCAKES WITH BERRIES 64
59. OMELET À LA MARGHERITA 65
60. OMELET WITH TOMATOES AND SPRING ONIONS 66
61. COCONUT CHIA PUDDING WITH BERRIES 66

62. Eel on Scrambled Eggs and Bread 67
63. Chia Seed Gel with Pomegranate and Nuts 68
64. Lavender Blueberry Chia Seed Pudding 68
65. Yogurt with Granola and Persimmon . 69
66. Fried Egg with Bacon 70
67. Whole Grain Bread and Avocado 70
68. Porridge with Walnuts 71
69. Zucchini Noodles with Creamy Avocado Pesto 72
70. Avocado Chicken Salad 72

CHAPTER 6: MAIN DISHES 74

71. Baked Ricotta with Pears 74
72. Herbed Wild Rice 75
73. Buffalo Chicken Sliders 75
74. High Protein Chicken Meatballs 76
75. Barley Risotto 77
76. Risotto with Green Beans, Sweet Potatoes, And Peas 77
77. Maple Lemon Tempeh Cubes 78
78. Bok Choy With Tofu Stir Fry 79
79. Three-Bean Medley 80
80. Herbed Garlic Black Beans 80
81. Quinoa with Vegetables 81
82. Pan-Fried Salmon 82
83. Mediterranean Chickpea Salad 82
84. Zucchini Salmon Salad 83
85. Greek Roasted Fish 83
86. Oregano Pork Mix 84
87. Simple Beef Roast 85
88. Pork and Peppers Chili 85
89. Chicken Breast Soup 86
90. Tomato Fish Bake 86
91. Warm Chorizo Chickpea Salad 87
92. Chicken Broccoli Salad with Avocado Dressing 88
93. Balsamic Beef and Mushrooms Mix 88
94. Garlicky Tomato Chicken Casserole 89
95. Fennel Wild Rice Risotto 90
96. Garlic Chicken Balls 90
97. Sliced Steak with Canadian Crust 91
98. Fork Tender Beef Goulash with Peppercorn & Sage 92
99. Mexican Chicken in Orange Juice 93
100. Chicken Sancho 94

CHAPTER 7: SIDES 96

101. Caramelized Onion Quesadilla 96
102. Roasted Garlic Potatoes 96
103. Asian Noodle Salad 97
104. Protein Pumpkin Spiced Donuts 98
105. Coconut Fat Bombs 99
106. Easy One-Pot Vegan Marinara 99
107. Sunflower Parmesan Cheese 100
108. Spicy Zucchini Slices 101
109. Cheddar Portobello Mushrooms 101
110. Salty Lemon Artichokes 102
111. Cheddar Potato Gratin 103
112. Parmesan Sweet Potato Casserole 103
113. Asparagus & Parmesan 104

CHAPTER 8: SEAFOOD 106

114. Shrimp Spring Rolls 106
115. Scallops with Tomato Cream Sauce ... 107
116. Sriracha & Honey Tossed Calamari 107
117. Southern Style Catfish with Green Beans 108
118. Roasted Salmon with Fennel Salad 109
119. Catfish with Cajun Seasoning 110
120. Sushi Roll 110
121. Garlic-Lime Shrimp Kebabs 111
122. Fish Finger Sandwich 112
123. Healthy Tuna Patties 112
124. Crab Cakes 113
125. Breaded Air Fried Shrimp with Bang-Bang Sauce 114
126. Crispy Fish Sandwich 115
127. Shrimp Egg Rolls 115

CHAPTER 9: VEGETABLES DISHES 118

128. Arugula Lentil Salad 118
129. Tomato Avocado Toast 119
130. Classic Tofu Salad 119
131. Moroccan Couscous Salad 120
132. Eggplant Curry 121
133. Asian Cabbage Rice 122
134. African Peanut Soup 123
135. Sweet Potato Soup 124
136. Roasted Garlic Wilted Spinach 125
137. Avocado Toast with Radish 126
138. Baba Ganoush 126
139. Black Bean Burgers 127

- 140. Chickpea Flour Pancake Fennel & Olive 128
- 141. Colorful Tabbouleh Salad 129
- 142. Easy Cauliflower Curry 130

CHAPTER 10: SOUPS AND SALADS 132
- 143. Swiss Cheese and Broccoli Soup 132
- 144. Tavern Soup..133
- 145. Broccoli Blue Cheese..........................133
- 146. Cream of Mushroom Soup 134
- 147. Olive Soup 135
- 148. Normandy Salad 136
- 149. Loaded Caesar Salad with Crunchy Chickpeas 137
- 150. Coleslaw Worth A Second Helping 138
- 151. Romaine Lettuce and Radicchios Mix ..139
- 152. Greek Salad 140
- 153. Asparagus and Smoked Salmon Salad 140
- 154. Shrimp Cobb Salad 141

CHAPTER 11: SNACKS...144
- 155. Bacon Cheeseburger 144
- 156. Cheeseburger Pie...............................145
- 157. Personal Pizza Biscuit 146
- 158. Chicken and Mushrooms....................146
- 159. Chicken Enchilada Bake 147
- 160. Jalapeno Lentil (Chickpea) Burgers + Avocado Mango Pico 148
- 161. Grandma's Rice 149
- 162. Baked Beef Zucchini...........................150
- 163. Baked Tuna with Asparagus 151
- 164. Lamb Stuffed Avocado 152
- 165. Sweet Almond Bites 152
- 166. Strawberry Cheesecake Minis 153
- 167. Cocoa Brownies..................................153
- 168. Chocolate Orange Bites 154
- 169. Caramel Cones 155
- 170. Cinnamon Bites 155
- 171. Sweet Chai Bites 156
- 172. Marinated Eggs 157

CHAPTER 12: DESSERTS.......................................158
- 173. Chocolate Bars...................................158
- 174. Blueberry Muffins 158
- 175. Chia Pudding......................................159
- 176. Avocado Pudding................................160
- 177. Peanut Butter Coconut Popsicle........160
- 178. Delicious Brownie Bites 161
- 179. Pumpkin Balls 161
- 180. Smooth Peanut Butter Cream............162
- 181. Vanilla Avocado Popsicles 162
- 182. Chocolate Popsicle 163
- 183. Raspberry Ice Cream 164
- 184. Chocolate Frosty................................164
- 185. Chocolate Almond Butter Brownie ...165
- 186. Peanut Butter Fudge 165

CHAPTER 13: SMOOTHIES 168
- 187. Creamy Raspberry Pomegranate Smoothie 168
- 188. Avocado Kale Smoothie 169
- 189. Apple Kale Cucumber Smoothie 169
- 190. Refreshing Cucumber Smoothie 170
- 191. Cauliflower Veggie Smoothie...............170
- 192. Soursop Smoothie 171
- 193. Tiramisu Shake 171
- 194. Vanilla Shake 172
- 195. Shamrock Shake.................................172
- 196. Coconut Smoothie 173
- 197. Vanilla Frappe 174
- 198. Pumpkin Frappe 174
- 199. Chocolate Frappe...............................175
- 200. Peppermint Mocha Shake 176

CHAPTER 14: OPTAVIA 28 DAYS MEAL PLAN AND SHOPPING LIST... 178
- 201. Shopping List Week 1 178
- Meal Plan Week 1 179
- Shopping List Week 2 180
- Meal Plan Week 2 181
- Shopping List Week 3 182
- Meal Plan Week 3 183
- Shopping List Week 4 184
- Meal Plan Week 4 185

CONCLUSION.. 186

LEAN AND GREEN DIET COOKBOOK:

Introduction

The Lean and Green Diet encourages people to limit the number of calories that they should take daily. To make this possible, dieters are motivated to choose healthier food items and meal replacements. But unlike other types of commercial diet regimens, the Lean and Green Diet comes in three different variations that one can choose according to their needs. Before we go in-depth, we should learn how to start, follow, and know the benefits of this Lean and Green diet plan.

How to Start This Diet?

The Lean and Green Diet has two unique phases, Initial and Maintenance Phases. Upon enrollment, you will be partnered and assigned to a diet coach to help you undertake all the necessary things to be a successful dieter. If you are wondering what steps you need to undertake while following the two phases, this guide will discuss that.

The initial phase is when people are encouraged to limit their calorie intake from 800 to 1,000 calories for the next 12 weeks or until the dieter loses 12 pounds. For this phase, dieters are encouraged to consume "Lean and Green" meals 5 to 7x daily. Moreover, dieters are also encouraged to consume one optional snack, including sugar-free gelatin, celery sticks, and 12 ounces of nuts.

On the other hand, the maintenance phase is implemented once you have already lost 12 pounds from your initial weight. During this phase, you can increase your calorie intake to 1,550 daily. This phase can last for six weeks. Moreover, you are also allowed to incorporate other foods such as whole grains, fruits, and low-fat dairy into your diet.

After the maintenance phase, you are now ready to follow your specific Lean and Green Diet plan. It is also when you need to consume not only "Lean and Green" meals but also fueling foods. The number of meals depends on the specific diet plan you choose. For instance, if you opt for the 3&3 Lean and Green plan, you need to consume three "Lean and Green" meals and three "Fuelings."

Initial Steps

Most people begin with the Optimum Weight 5&1 Diet for weight reduction, an 800 to 1,000 calorie routine that will help you lose 12 pounds over 12 weeks. You are expected to consume one meal every 2-3 hours and have moderate activity for half an hour on some days of the week. In general, no more than 100 grams of carbs are given per day by the Fuelings and portions. As Lean and Green coaches get paid on commission, you will order these meals from your coach's specific page.

Lean and Green meals aim to be high in protein and low in carbs. One meal provides 5, 7(cooked) ounces of lean protein, three portions of vegetables mostly non-starchy, and up to 2 portions of good fats. This schedule also involves one extra snack a day (which the coach would accept), three celery sticks, half a cup of sugar-free gelatin, or a half-ounce of nuts are plan-approved treats. Bear in mind that the 5&1 Strategy does not allow alcohol intake.

Maintenance Phase

When you achieve the target weight, you begin a six-week maintenance period, which entails steadily raising calories to 1,550 calories but not more than that each day and incorporating low-fat dairy, whole grains, and fruits in a larger range of foods.

You are expected to switch over to the "Ideal Wellness" 3&3 Schedule after six weeks, which involves 3 "Lean & Green" meals and 3 Fuels every day with regular Lean and Green coaching. Many who had continuous progress on the platform can be qualified as a coach for Lean and Green.

How to Follow the Lean and Green Diet?

While the Lean and Green Diet is all about delivering weight loss to its dieters, dieters' success still largely depends on how they approach this particular diet regimen. Thus, if you want to become successful, below are the tips that you should do while following the Lean and Green Diet:

- To follow the diet first off, you must start with a conversation with the Lean and Green diet coach to determine which Lean and Green plan is best suited for your goal. It could be weight loss or weight maintenance and make yourself familiar with the program.

- Opt for foods that are cooked using healthy cooking methods. Healthy cooking methods include baking, grilling, poaching, and broiling. Avoid frying your foods as cooking oil increases the calorie content of your food.

- Portion sizes of your food should follow the Lean and Green recommendations. It means that the portion sizes refer to the cooked weight and not the raw weight of the ingredients that you are using.

- Opt for foods rich in Omega-3 fatty acids such as tuna, salmon, mackerel, trout, herring, and many other cold-water fishes. Omega-3 fatty acids contribute to lowering inflammation in the body.

- Choose meatless alternatives such as tofu and tempeh. They are rich in proteins but not too much in calories.

- Following the program at all costs, even if you are dining out. It means that you have to consume healthy meals when you eat out and make sure that you stay away from alcohol.

The Benefits of Lean and Green Diet

Easy to Follow

With the Lean and Green diet, you have to rely on prepackaged fuelings and be required to cook your lean and green recipe meal, which will only be once per day if you are on the 5&1 plan, and it doesn't take long to get prepared.

For any plan you subscribed to, you will get meal logs together with sample meal plans, which can make things easier for you. You will also get a list of food options with specific recipes. If you feel not to cook, you can buy packaged meals, otherwise known as Flavors of Home, as a replacement for your Lean and Green meals.

It Can Improve Blood Pressure

Taking part in the Lean and Green Diet program can improve your blood pressure since you will be consuming less sodium and shed weight. With the Lean and Green meals, you will have the option of consuming less than 2,300 mg of sodium in a day — if you choose the Lean and Green meals with low sodium options. Consuming less than 2,300 mg of salt daily will positively affect your blood pressure. That is why many health organizations such as the United States Department of Agriculture (USDA), American Heart Association, Institute of Medicine, and other health institutions recommend it. It is pertinent to note that higher sodium intake in salt-sensitive individuals can result in heart disease and increased blood pressure risk.

Provides Ongoing Support

You will have access to a certified health coach either in the weight maintenance or weight loss programs. Current research proves that having a counselor or lifestyle coach can positively impact your weight loss or maintenance.

No Counting of Calories, Points, Or Carbs

Once you are on the diet program, you are expected to feed on the Lean and Green Fuelings with Lean and Green meals, and as such, you do not have to count your calories, points, or carbs intake.

Nutritionally Sound

Even though you will be feeding on meals that are very low in calories and carbs, they still meet the nutritional requirements; hence, you do not have to panic about nutrition deficiency.

Lose Weight Rapidly

With the Lean and Green diet, you are sure to lose weight within four weeks of being on the program once you follow your plan's guidelines, and you keep to your coach's advice.

LEAN AND GREEN DIET COOKBOOK:

CHAPTER 1:

Fundamentals of Lean and Green Program

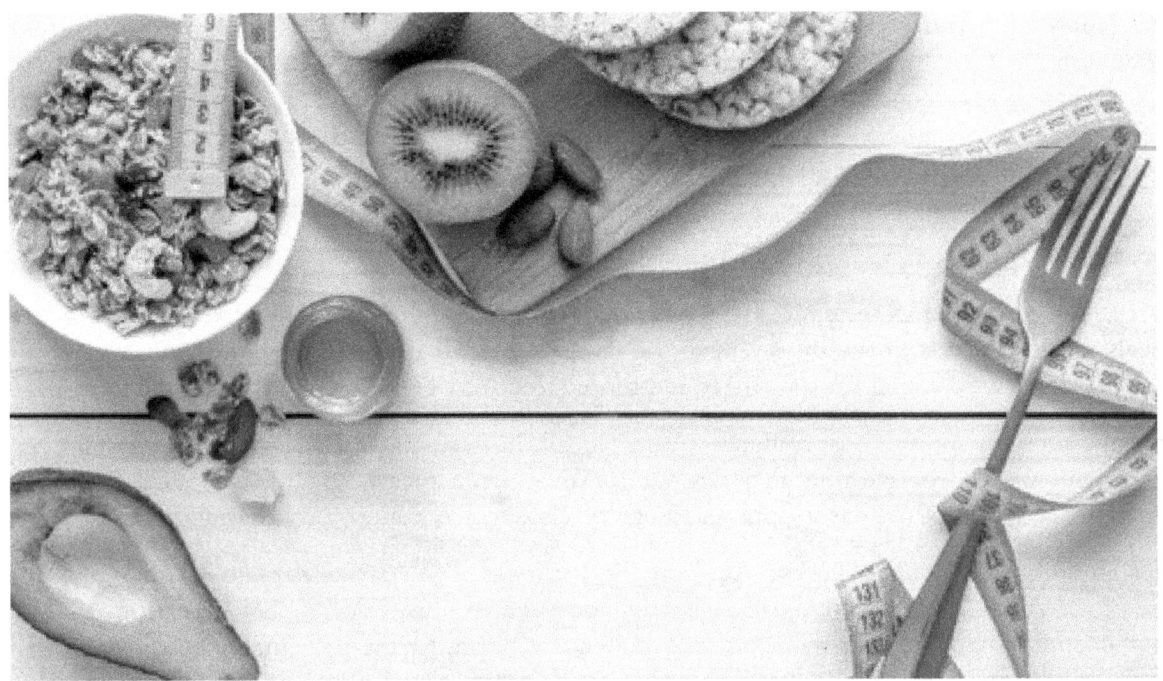

The Medifast, along with the Lean and Green diet, is one of the most effective diet plans for people who want to lose weight. The module of programs in the Medifast Diet is very varied and is perfect for many individuals. It is essentially a very restricted diet plan that can be undergone for a period ranging between 4-6 weeks. It has been beneficial for many individuals in losing and maintaining their weight for many years.

The plan is aimed at meeting the nutritional needs of a person and keeping him healthy. The program is known to boost the metabolism and help a person' tone' his or her muscles. The program keeps one's body fit and healthy.

Many people have raised questions about the Lean and Green Diet Program. The Lean and Green diet can be explained as a weight loss plan, which can be based on eating several meals per day called fuelings. All these mini-meals provisioned are supposed to be contented for you and fill you up and help you shed many pounds. For those accustomed to Medifast meal supplements, Lean and Green is essential because it's an updated version that comes with an excellent meal plan.

There are various variants of the Lean and Green diet that one may receive. In this part, we're going to talk about the fundamentals Lean and Green program that you can use and help you while you embraced this beneficial lifestyle:

5&1 Lean and Green Diet Plan

5&1 Lean and Green diet plan is essentially just a modification of the 3&1 that differs in a few essential steps. If your weight falls in a range of 2-10 pounds, you should choose the 5&1 Lean and Green diet. As you realize, you will be having 5 Lean and Green meals per day.

It is highly advised that you consume just five items per day, and you are free to pick any of them. The reason to have five instead of 3 is that it gives you more liberty of choosing the kind of food that makes you feel full and happy. You can choose to run to the market and purchase items that you want, or you can consume the fat-burning foods available on the official site. The Optavia program offers you cooking guides regarding the items that you want to avoid with your diet plan and the items you could consume with it.

4&2&1 Lean and Green Diet Plan

Just a 4 & 2 & 1 plan is the same as 5 & 1, but instead of five meals, you will be having only four meals. But all the rest of the steps remain the same as in 5&1. It is highly recommended to opt for 4&2&1 if you are looking for a stronger and more effective weight loss plan.

It is the simplest and the least difficult one among all the variants of the Lean and Green diet plan. Here your dietary routine only includes 4 Lean and Green meals, and the last meal is optional. Since the last meal of the day is optional, it can be chosen according to your convenience.

It is highly recommended that you consume the last meal of the day, either late evening or early in the morning. It is because, alongside sleeping, you need to burn calories. There is a lot of activity in the body while sleeping that you take in fewer calories. Thus it is highly recommended to consume the last meal of the day earlier. You will feel more energetic to have a good workout session.

3&3 Lean and Green Diet Plan

3&3 Lean and Green diet plan is a modification of the "4 & 2 & 1 Lean and Green diet plan. Your caloric intake per day will be 1000 calories against 1200 that you are supposed to have in the 4&2&1 Lean and Green diet plan.

This plan is also more flexible as you can choose the meals as per your craving. It is highly recommended that you consume your three meals in intervals of 3 hours. It would be the best way to feel full. It should be taken for granted that you reduce the number of carbohydrates and replace them with fat.

Many people are associated with following such a diet plan and feel full all through the day. Thus it is highly recommended to follow it.

CHAPTER 2:

How Does Lean and Green Work?

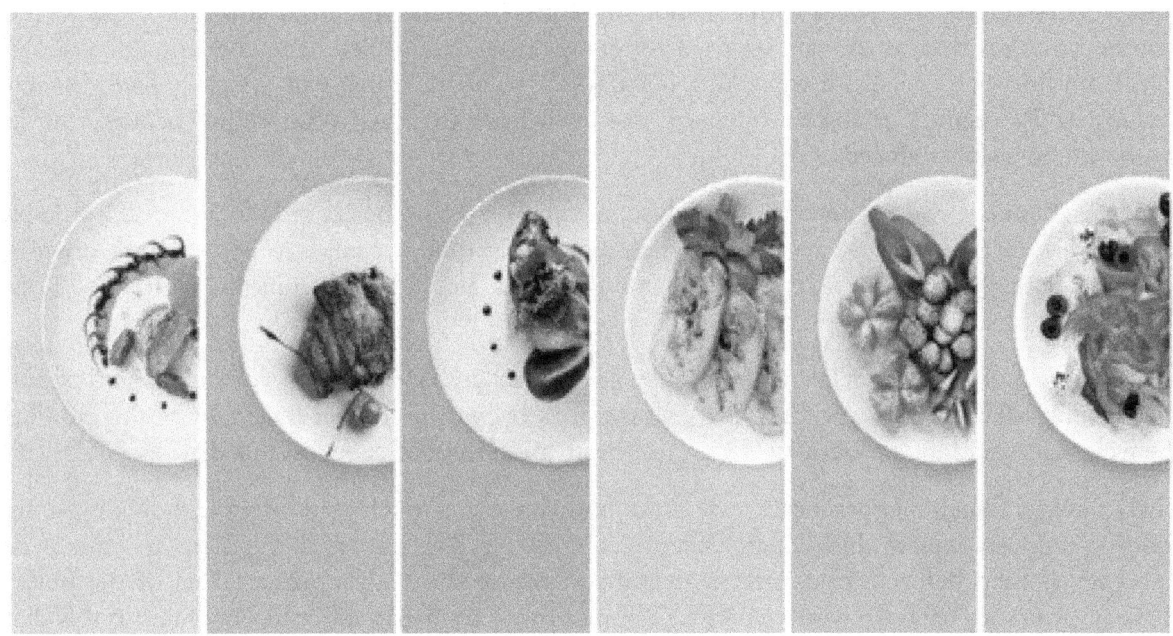

We will now talk about how this diet works and how your body transitions from one way to another. Before, the Lean and Green diet was used mainly to lower the incidence of seizures in epileptic children.

People wanted to check out how the Lean and Green diet would work with an entirely healthy person as things usually go. This diet's primary purpose is to make your body switch from how it used to function to an entirely new way of creating energy, keeping you healthy and alive.

How Lean and Green Works?

Once you start following the Lean and Green Diet, you will notice that things are changing, first and foremost, in your mind. Before, carbohydrates were your main body 'fuel' and were used to create glucose so that your brain could function. Now you no longer feed yourself with them.

In the beginning, most people feel odd because their usual food is off the table. When your menu consists of more fats and proteins, it is natural to think that something is missing.

Your brain alarms you that you haven't eaten enough and sends you signals that you are hungry. It is literally "panicking" and telling you that you are starving, which is not correct. You get to eat, and you get to eat plenty of good food, but not carbs.

This condition usually arises during the first day or two. Afterward, people get used to their new eating habits. Once the brain "realizes" that carbs are no longer an option, it will focus on "finding" another abundant energy source: in this case, fats.

Not only are your food rich in fats, but your body contains stored fats in large amounts. As you consume more fats and fewer carbs, your body "runs" on the fats, both consumed and stored. The best thing is that, as the fats are used for energy, they are burned. It is how you get a double gain from this diet. Usually, it will take a few days of consuming low-carb meals before you start seeing visible weight loss results. You will not even have to check your weight because the fat layers will be visibly reduced.

This diet requires you to lower your daily consumption of carbs to only 20 grams. For most people, this transition from a regular carb-rich diet can be quite a challenge. Most people are used to eating bread, pasta, rice, dairy products, sweets, soda, alcohol, and fruits, so quitting all these foods might be challenging.

However, this is all in your head. If you manage to win the "battle" with your mind and endure the diet for a few days, you will see that as time goes by, you no longer have cravings at all. Plus, the weight loss and the fat burn will be a great motivation to continue with this diet.

The Lean and Green diet practically makes the body burn fats much faster than carbohydrates; the foods you consume with this diet are exceptionally rich in fats. Carbs will be there, too but at far lower levels than before. Foods rich in carbohydrates are the body's primary fuel or the brain's food. (Our bodies turn carbs into glucose.) Because there are hardly any carbohydrates in this diet, the body will have to find a substitute source of energy to keep itself alive.

Many people who don't truly need to lose weight and are completely healthy still choose to follow the Lean and Green diet because it is a great way to keep their meals balanced. This lifestyle is also an excellent way to cleanse the body of toxins, processed foods, sugars, and unnecessary carbs. The combination of these things is usually the main reason for heart failure, some cancers, diabetes, cholesterol, or obesity.

If you ask a nutritionist about this diet, they will recommend it without a doubt. So, if you feel like cleansing your body and starting a diet that will keep you healthy, well-fed, and slender, perhaps the Lean and Green diet should be your primary choice.

And what is the best thing about it besides the fact that you will balance your weight and lower the risk of many diseases? There is no yo-yo effect. The Lean and Green diet can be followed forever and has no side effects. It does not restrict you from pursuing it for a few weeks or a month. Once you get your body used to Lean and Green foods, you will not think about going back to the old ways of eating your meals.

CHAPTER 3:

Recommended Food That Are Allowed and Not Allowed

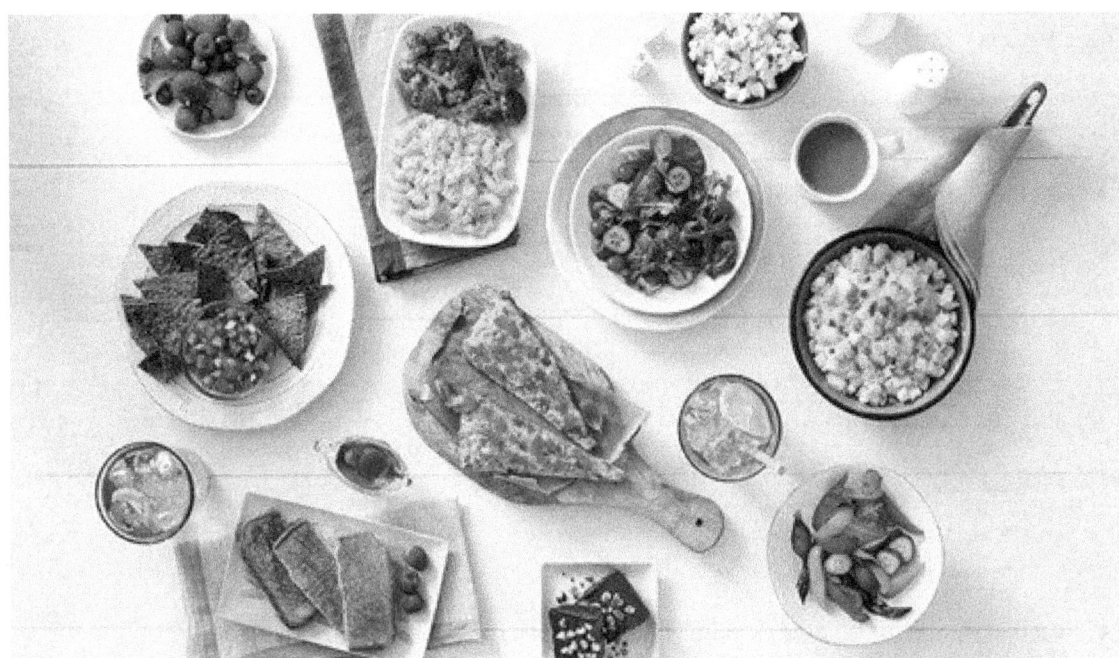

There are so many foods that you can eat while following the Lean and Green Diet. However, you must know these foods by heart. It is especially true if you are just new to this diet, and you have to strictly follow the 5&1 Lean and Green Diet Plan. Thus, this section is dedicated to the types of foods you can eat and cannot follow this diet regimen.

Foods That Are Allowed

There are several categories of foods that can be eaten under this diet regimen. This section will break down the Lean and Green foods you can eat while following this diet regime.

Leanest Foods

These foods are considered the leanest as it has only up to 4 grams of total fat. Moreover, dieters should eat a 7-ounce cooked portion of these foods. Consume these foods with 1 healthy fat serving:

- Fish: Flounder, cod, haddock, grouper, Mahi, tilapia, tuna (yellowfin fresh or canned), and wild catfish.

- Shellfish: Scallops, lobster, crabs, shrimp

- Game meat: Elk, deer, buffalo

- Ground turkey or other meat: Should be 98% lean

- Meatless alternatives:14 egg whites, 2 cups egg substitute, 5 ounces' seitan, 1 ½ cups 1% cottage cheese, and 12 ounces non-fat 0% Greek yogurt

Leaner Foods

These foods contain 5 to 9 grams of total fat. Consume these foods with one healthy fat serving. Make sure to consume only 6 ounces of a cooked portion of these foods daily:

- Fish: Halibut, trout, and swordfish

- Chicken: White meat such as breasts as long as the skin is removed

- Turkey: Ground turkey as long as it is 95% to 97% lean.

- Meatless options: 2 whole eggs plus four egg whites, two whole eggs plus one cup egg substitute, 1 ½ cups 2% cottage cheese, and 12 ounces' low fat 2% plain Greek yogurt

Lean Foods

These are foods that contain 10g to 20g total fat. When consuming these foods, there should be no serving of healthy fat. These include the following:

- Fish: Tuna (Bluefin steak), salmon, herring, farmed catfish, and mackerel

- Lean beef: Ground, steak, and roast

- Lamb: All cuts

- Pork: Pork chops, pork tenderloin, and all parts. Make sure to remove the skin

- Ground turkey and other meats:85% to 94% lean

- Chicken: Any dark meat

- Meatless options:15 ounces' extra-firm tofu, three whole eggs (up to two times per week), 4 ounces reduced-fat skim cheese, 8 ounces' part-skim ricotta cheese, and 5 ounces' tempeh

Healthy Fat Servings

Healthy fat servings are allowed under this diet. They should contain 5 grams of fat and less than grams of carbohydrates. Regardless of what type of Lean and Green Diet plan you follow, make sure that you add between 0 and 2 healthy fat servings daily. Below are the different healthy fat servings that you can eat:

- 1 teaspoon oil (any kind of oil)
- 1 tablespoon low carbohydrate salad dressing
- 2 tablespoons reduced-fat salad dressing
- 5 to 10 black or green olives
- 1 ½ ounce avocado
- 1/3-ounce plain nuts including peanuts, almonds, pistachios
- 1 tablespoon plain seeds such as chia, sesame, flax, and pumpkin seeds
- ½ tablespoon regular butter, mayonnaise, and margarine

Green Foods

This part will talk about the green servings you still need to consume while following the Lean and Green Diet Plan. These include all kinds of vegetables categorized from lower, moderate, and high in carbohydrate content. One serving of vegetables should be at ½ cup unless otherwise specified.

Lower Carbohydrate - These are vegetables that contain low amounts of carbohydrates. If you are following the 5&1 Lean and Green Diet plan, then these vegetables are right for you:

- A cup of green leafy vegetables such as collard greens (raw), lettuce (green leaf, iceberg, butterhead, and romaine), spinach (raw), mustard greens, spring mix, bok choy (raw), and watercress.
- ½ cup of vegetables including cucumbers, celery, radishes, white mushroom, sprouts (mung bean, alfalfa), arugula, turnip greens, escarole, nopales, Swiss chard (raw), jalapeno, and bok choy (cooked).

Moderate Carbohydrate - These are vegetables that contain moderate amounts of carbohydrates. Below are the types of vegetables that can be consumed in moderation:

- ½ cup of any of the following vegetables such as asparagus, cauliflower, a fennel bulb, eggplant, portabella mushrooms, kale, cooked spinach, summer squash (zucchini and scallop).

Higher Carbohydrates - Foods that are under this category contain a high amount of starch. Make sure to consume limited amounts of these vegetables.

- ½ cup of the following vegetables like chayote squash, red cabbage, broccoli, cooked collard and mustard greens, green or wax beans, kohlrabi, kabocha squash, cooked leeks, any peppers, okra, raw scallion, summer squash such as straight neck and crookneck, tomatoes, spaghetti squash, turnips, jicama, cooked Swiss chard, and hearts of palm.

Foods That Are Not Allowed

There are many types of foods that are not allowed for the Lean and Green Diet Plan. These foods either contain high amounts of fats or carbohydrates that can contribute to weight gain. Below are the types of foods that are not allowed under this particular diet:

- Fried foods
- Alcohol
- Milk
- Cheese
- Fruit juice
- Soda and other sweetened beverages
- Refined grains like pasta, white rice, and white bread

CHAPTER 4:

Lean and Green Recipes

1. Adobo Sirloin

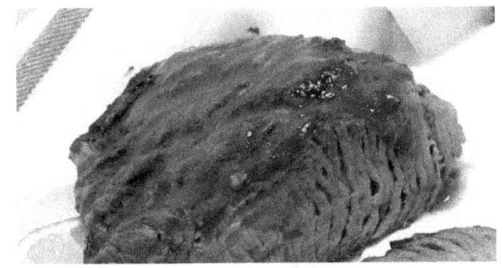

Preparation time: 15 minutes

Cooking time: 5 minutes

Servings: 2

Level of difficulty: Normal

Category: Leaner

Ingredients:

- 1 lime juice
- 1 tablespoon chopped garlic
- 1 tablespoon of dried oregano
- 1 teaspoon cumin
- 2 tablespoons of finely chopped chipotle chilies in adobo sauce plus 2 spoonsful of sauce
- 4 sirloin steaks (6-ounce), trimmed with fat
- Salt and black chili pepper, to taste

Directions:

1. Combine the lime juice, garlic, oregano, cumin, chilies, and adobo sauce in a small cup. Healthy balance to blend.
2. Season with salt and pepper to taste. Put steaks with adobo marinade into a big Ziploc container, then seal tightly and cover with a shake. Refrigerate, trembling slightly, for at least 2 hours.
3. Prepare a grill to high heat. Cover the barbecue grills loosely with a cooking spray. Once the grill is heated, cook steaks on each side for about 4 to 5 minutes until the desired doneness. Give the steaks 10 minutes to rest and serve.

Nutrition:

Calories: 213

Carbs: 4g

Fat: 7g

Protein: 37g

2. Beef Stroganoff

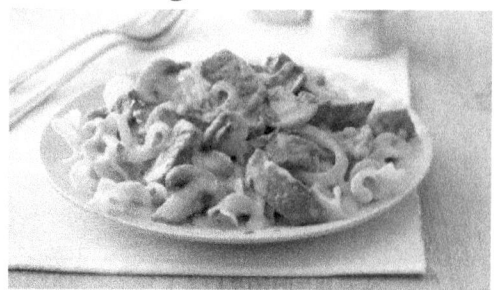

Preparation time: 15 minutes

Cooking time: 30 minutes

Servings: 2

Level of difficulty: Normal

Category: Lean

Ingredients:

- Salt and black chili pepper, to taste
- 8 oz. egg noodles
- Trimmed with fat and a sliced pound of beef
- 1 tablespoon of extra virgin olive oil
- ½ medium sliced onion
- 4 ounces of white, sliced mushrooms
- 1 tablespoon of cornstarch
- 1 (10.5-ounce) can condense, divided beef broth
- 1 teaspoon Dijon mustard
- 1 clove of garlic, minced and peeled
- 3 spoonsful of white wine
- ½ tablespoon Worcestershire sauce
- 2 spoonsful of low-fat sour cream
- 2 tablespoons cream cheese with reduced-fat

Directions:

1. Pick up a big pot of lightly salted water over high heat to a boil. Cook noodles as indicated on the box. Drain, and set aside.

2. In the meantime, season the beef with salt and pepper—heat oil over medium heat in a large skillet. Add beef; brown on all sides, then force one side of the saucepan.

3. Put the onion plus mushrooms and cook for around 3 to 5 minutes until tender. Move beef to the left. Combine cornstarch and 2 tablespoons of cold beef broth in a small tub. Apply to the skillet and whisk to deglaze with the juices in the pan.

4. Pour the remainder of the beef broth down. Bring to a boil, with regular stirring. Reduce to low heat and stir in mustard, garlic, wine, and sauce from Worcestershire. Cover with a tight cap and cook for 10 minutes.

5. Stir in sour cream and cream cheese, two minutes until the beef is cooked. Remove and allow the beef to finish the sauce cooking. Let meat rest for five minutes and serve.

Nutrition:

Calories: 139 Carbs: 7g Fat: 6g

Protein: 15g

3. Savory Burgers

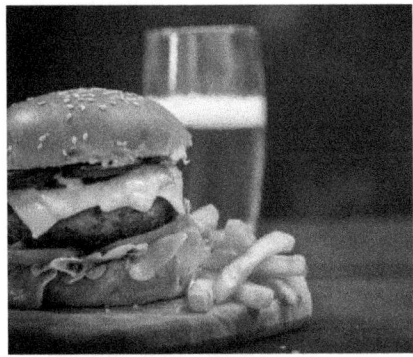

Preparation time: 15 minutes

Cooking time: 15 minutes

Servings: 4

Level of difficulty: Normal

Category: Lean

Ingredients:

- 1 ½ pound 92 percent lean ground beef
- 4 tablespoons Dijon mustard
- Salt and black chili pepper, to taste
- ½ cup of low carb ketchup
- ½ cup mayonnaise light
- 1 tablespoon of red vinegar
- 2 teaspoons Worcestershire sauce
- 4 whole-wheat hamburger buns
- 4 pickles sandwich slices, halved

Directions:

1. Prepare a grill to heat high. Cover the barbecue grills loosely with a cooking spray.
2. Combine beef, mustard, salt, and pepper in one large bowl. Form into 4 patties of the same size and grill the patties for 5 to 6 minutes per side.
3. Meanwhile, mix the ketchup, mayonnaise, vinegar, and Worcestershire sauce in a small bowl.
4. Cut the buns in half and place on the grill toast side down until a light golden brown, about 10 seconds. Put hamburgers on buns, and top with sauce and pickles. Serve.

Nutrition:

Calories: 415 Carbs: 32g

Fat: 12g Protein: 41g

4. Beef Lo Mein

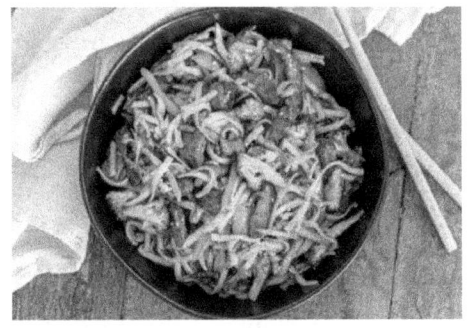

Preparation time: 15 minutes

Cooking time: 20 minutes

Servings: 2

Level of difficulty: Normal

Category: Lean

Ingredients:

- Salt, enough to taste

- 2 oz. whole-wheat spaghetti
- 1 tablespoon of sesame oil
- 1 sirloin steak (6-ounce), fat trimmed and cut into strips
- 1/4 cup of fresh pea pods, cut
- 1/4 cup of broccoli blossoms
- 1 ½ cup shredded carrots
- Scallion, hammered
- 1/8 red pepper flakes in a teaspoon
- ½ clove of garlic, minced and peeled
- 2 tablespoons soy sauce with less sodium
- ½ teaspoon of fresh ginger peeled and grated
- 1 teaspoon of sesame seeds

Directions:

1. Boil a pot of lightly salted water up over high heat. Cook spaghetti as instructed on the box. Drain, and set aside.
2. In the meantime, over medium-high heat, steam oil in a wok or large skillet. Connect the beef and stir-fry for about 4 to 6 minutes until brown. Remove, and set aside from the pan.
3. Add snow peas, broccoli, cabbage, scallion, and garlic—Stir-fry for 2 to 3 minutes. Add soy sauce, ginger, reserved noodles, and beef to taste. Mix nice and cook until hot. Remove wok from heat and garnish with sesame seeds to stir-fry.

Nutrition:

Calories: 440

Carbs: 65g

Fat: 7g

Protein: 28g

5. Beef Lasagna

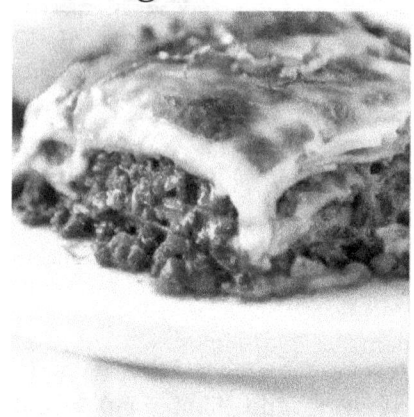

Preparation time: 15 minutes

Cooking time: 60 minutes

Servings: 2

Level of difficulty: Normal

Category: Lean

Ingredients:

- 2 tablespoons extra virgin olive oil
- ½ pound 92 percent lean ground beef
- ½ little onion, sliced
- ½ teaspoon of dried oregano
- 1 cup with tomato sauce

- 1 cup cheese with low-fat ricotta
- 1 tablespoon rubbed Parmesan cheese
- 6 lasagna noodles on no-boil
- 1 zucchini, thinly sliced

Directions:

1. Preheat to 350°F on the burner. Warm oil over medium to high heat in a big, non-stick skillet. Add beef, onion, oregano, and pepper to the pan, using a wooden spoon to cut the meat into small pieces.
2. Cook, constantly stirring for 6 to 8 minutes until the meat is thoroughly cooked. Remove from heat and whisk in tomato sauce, bring to a boil.
3. Blend ricotta and Parmesan in a small tub. Layer ingredients in a 9-inch by 13-inch baking dish to create lasagna: begin with 1/2 cup sauce, 2 noodles, and ½ cup cheese mixture.
4. Put an extra ½ cup sauce and half a slice of zucchini. Continue layering with 2 noodles, ½ cup cheese mixture, ½ cup sauce, and remaining portions of zucchini. Top with ½ cup sauce remaining and 2 noodles leftover.
5. Cover the platter with foil, and bake 30 minutes in the oven. Remove foil and bake for another 15 minutes. Remove from the oven, and let the lasagna sit to eat for at least 10 minutes before cutting.

Nutrition:

Calories: 480

Carbs: 28g

Fat: 22g

Protein: 39g

6. Teriyaki Sirloin Steaks

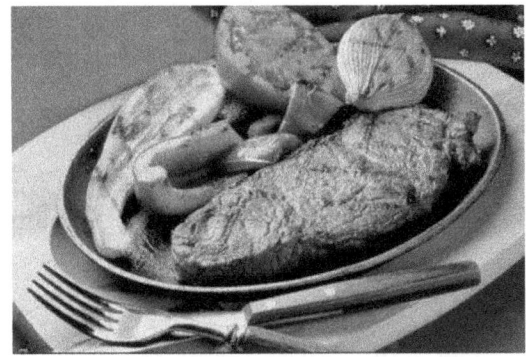

Preparation time: 2 hours & 10 minutes

Cooking time: 10 minutes

Servings: 4

Level of difficulty: Normal

Category: Lean

Ingredients:

- 1/3 cup soy sauce, less sodium
- 2 spoonsful of molasses
- 2 teaspoons Dijon mustard
- Garlic, roasted and minced
- 2 tbsp ginger, peeled and grated
- 4 (6-ounce) sirloin steaks, fat
- Salt and black pepper ground to taste

Directions:

1. Add soy sauce, molasses, Dijon mustard, garlic, and ginger in a small cup. Whisk in until mixed.
2. In a large Ziploc bag, put steaks, season with salt and pepper, and pour in the marinade. Seal firmly, shake to seal, and refrigerate steaks, shaking periodically for at least 2 hours.
3. Prepare a grill to high heat. Cover the barbecue grills loosely with a cooking spray. Once the grill is heated, grill steaks untouched for 4 minutes.
4. Use tongs to turn the steaks and grill for another 4 to 6 minutes, depending on the doneness you want. Let the steaks rest and serve for 10 minutes.

Nutrition:

Calories: 260 Carbs: 7g

Fat: 12g Protein: 35g

7. Salisbury Steak

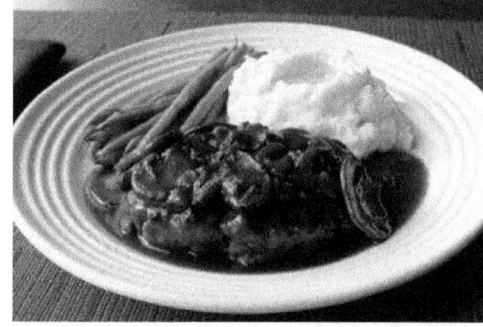

Preparation time: 15 minutes

Cooking time: 15 minutes

Servings: 5

Level of difficulty: Normal

Category: Lean

Ingredients:

- 3 cups of sliced white mushrooms, split
- 1-pound 92 percent lean ground beef
- ¼ cup regular breadcrumbs
- Egg whites or 6 spoonful of liquid egg white replacement
- ¼ cup 2% milk
- ¼ cup of dried thyme
- 2 tablespoons of low-carbon ketchup, split
-
- 1 (12-ounce) fat-free gravy beef jar

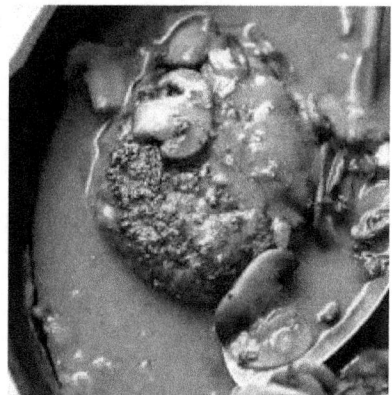

Directions:

1. Chop 1 cup of mushrooms good and then save the remaining sliced mushrooms for later. Combine sliced mushrooms, ground beef,

breadcrumbs, egg whites, honey, thyme, and 1 liter of ketchup in a big dish. Mix until well blended.

2. Form into 5 oval patties, roughly ½-inch thick. Cover a big, non-stick skillet over medium-high heat with cooking spray and warm. Add the patties, cook until both sides brown, around 2 to 3 minutes per hand.

3. Add the remaining 2 cups of mushrooms to the pan, the remaining two ketchup spoons, and gravy onto the pan. Boil the blend; reduce heat to medium.

4. Cover and allow to simmer within 5-10 minutes until thoroughly cooked patties. Serve gravy on patties.

Nutrition:

Calories: 186

Carbs: 6g

Fat: 10g

Protein: 17g

8. Beef and Chicken Sausage-Stuffed Mini Peppers

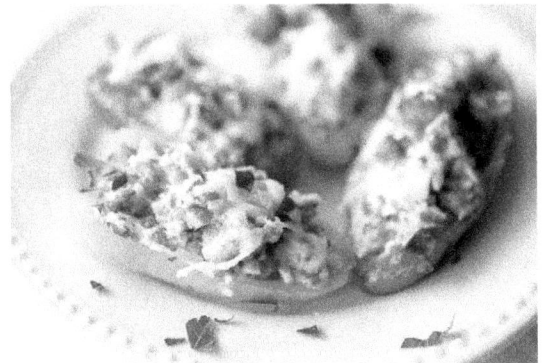

Preparation time: 15 minutes

Cooking time: 32 minutes

Servings: 2

Level of difficulty: Normal

Category: Lean

Ingredients:

- 1 tablespoon of extra virgin olive oil
- 1 cup of shredded onion
- ¼-pound 92 percent lean ground beef
- 1/4 pound of chicken sausage
- ½ cup medium-grain cooked rice
- ¼ cup scallions hacked
- 1 teaspoon of sweet paprika
- ½ teaspoon cayenne chili pepper
- 1 teaspoon of dried oregano
- Salt and black chili pepper, to taste
- 24 mini peppers, tops and seeds removed

Directions:

1. Warm oven to 400 F. Heat oil over medium heat in a large skillet. Add onion, stir regularly, and cook until lightly brown and translucent.

2. Take off heat and move onion to a medium cup. Put beef, bacon, rice, scallions, paprika, cayenne, oregano, salt, and pepper into the dish. Healthy mix.

3. Use a spoon to stem the mixture into each pepper's cavity. Add peppers to a shallow pan and cover with foil made of aluminum. Bake the peppers for 30 minutes, or until they are crispy and crusty.

Nutrition:

Calories: 320

Carbs: 15g

Fat: 17g

Protein: 28g

9. Grilled Rosemary Lamb Chops

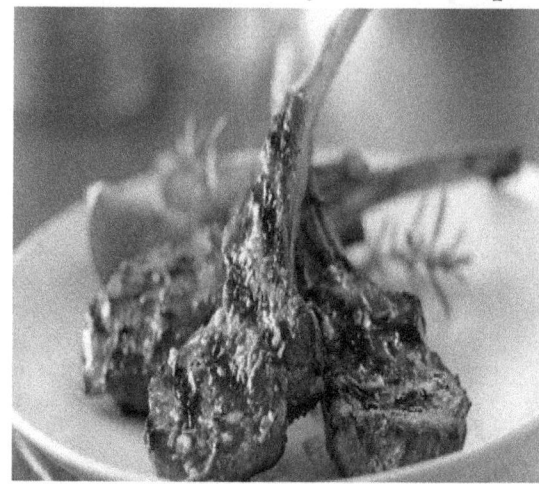

Preparation time: 15 minutes

Cooking time: 8 minutes

Servings: 4

Level of difficulty: Normal

Category: Lean

Ingredients:

- 1 tablespoon of extra virgin olive oil
- 1 lemon juice
- 3 garlic cloves, peeled and chopped
- 1 tablespoon fresh rosemary leaves black pepper and salt to taste
- 8 lamb chops (4-ounce), fat trimmed

Directions:

1. Mix the olive oil, lemon juice, garlic, and rosemary in a small bowl.
2. In a large Ziploc bag, put lamb chops, season with salt and pepper, and pour in the marinade. Seal firmly, shake to coat, and refrigerate lamb for at least 1 hour, shaking periodically, until overnight.
3. Prepare a grill to medium-high heat. Cover the barbecue grills loosely with a cooking spray.
4. Reject marinade. Once the grill is heated, roast the lamb on each side for 4 minutes. Let the chopped lamb rest 10 minutes and serve 2 chops per person.

Nutrition:

Calories: 123

Carbs: 2g

Fat: 8g

Protein: 12g

10. Honey-Mustard Leg of Lamb

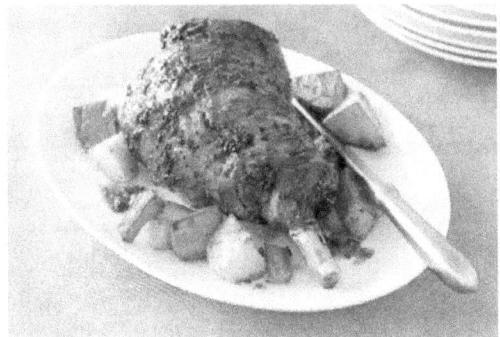

Preparation time: 15 minutes

Cooking time: 1 hour & 5 minutes

Servings: 2

Level of difficulty: Normal

Category: Lean

Ingredients:

- ¼ cup honey
- 2 tablespoons Dijon mustard
- 2 tablespoons chopped leaves of fresh thyme
- garlic cloves, peeled and grated
- salt and black chili pepper, to taste
- 5 lb. leg of lamb

Directions:

1. Preheat to 450°F on the burner. Stir honey, mustard, thyme, garlic, salt, and pepper in a small cup.
2. Put the lamb in a roasting pan over a rack. Rub the mixture of honey and mustard onto the lamb. 20 minutes to bake in the oven.
3. Reduce heat to 400°F, and add another 45 minutes to roast the lamb. For medium-rare doneness, the internal temperature on a meat thermometer should be at least 140°F. Until carving, let the lamb rest for 10 minutes.

Nutrition:

Calories: 239

Carbs: 1g

Fat: 19g

Protein: 18g

11. Pork Chops Braised with Oranges

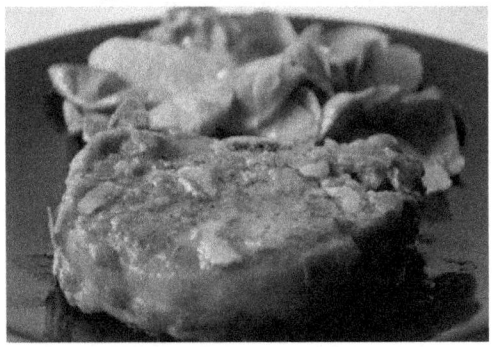

Preparation time: 15 minutes

Cooking time: 30 minutes

Servings: 2

Level of difficulty: Normal

Category: Leaner

Ingredients:

- 4 (6-ounce) boneless chops of pork trimmed with fat

- Salt and black pepper, to taste
- 1 (11-ounce) oranges with mandarin, drained
- ½ spoonful of ground cloves

Directions:

1. Season pork chops with salt and pepper, pressing into meat for seasoning.
2. Spray a large skillet over medium-high heat, cooking spray, and cover. Add each pork chop to the saucepan and sauté on both sides until golden brown. Pour oranges over the end, and sprinkle with cloves on the pork chops.
3. Cover with a tight lid over the pan and reduce heat to a minimum. Braise for about 20 to 25 minutes until meat is cooked through.

Nutrition:

Calories: 247 Carbs: 13g

Fat: 4g Protein: 38g

12. Plum Sauce-Glazed Pork Chops

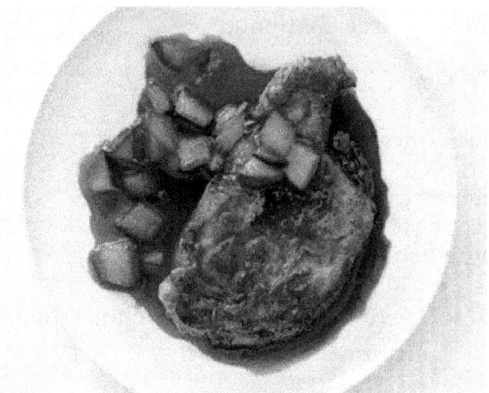

Preparation time: 15 minutes

Cooking time: 10 minutes

Servings: 2

Level of difficulty: Normal

Category: Leaner

Ingredients:

- 6-ounce bone-free pork chops, fat trimmed
- ¼ teaspoon of salt
- ¼ teaspoon black chili pepper
- ¼ cup Chinese plum sauce
- 4 teaspoons yellow mustard

Directions:

1. Season with salt and pepper to the pork chops. Cover a big, non-stick skillet over medium-high heat with cooking spray and warm.
2. Add pork chops to the skillet, cook until the center is no longer pink, around 3 minutes per hand.
3. Combine plum sauce and mustard into a small tub. Brown the mixture and serve on top of each pork chop.

Nutrition:

Calories: 150

Carbs: 21g

Fat: 6g

Protein: 2g

13. Dijon and Sage-Coated Pork Tenderloin

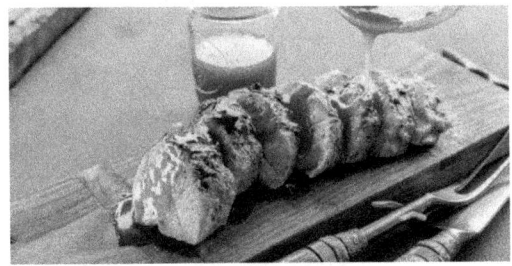

Preparation time: 15 minutes

Cooking time: 25 minutes

Servings: 3

Level of difficulty: Normal

Category: Lean

Ingredients:

- 1 lb. pork tenderloin, fat-cut
- 1 tablespoon extra-virgin olive oil
- Salt and black pepper to taste
- 2 tablespoons Dijon mustard
- 2 garlic cloves, peeled and chopped
- 1 tablespoon of fresh sage, finely chopped

Directions:

1. Preheat to 375°F on the burner. Cover with a cooking spray, and set aside a shallow baking pan. Pat the pork dry using paper towels and season with salt and pepper.
2. Warm oil over high heat in a big, non-stick skillet. When the pan is hot but not yet smoking, add pork, turning periodically for around 4 minutes until browned on all sides. Switch to the baking pan to prepare.
3. Cover with mustard and garlic over the pork and sage. Roast in the middle rack of the oven until a 2-inch instant-read thermometer inserted diagonally into the meat registers 145°F, around 20 minutes.
4. Move pork to a cutting board and cover with foil made of aluminum. Until slicing and serving, let the pork rest for 10 minutes.

Nutrition:

Calories: 172 Carbs: 1g Fat: 6g Protein: 26g

14. Smothered Cajun Pork Chops with Tomatoes

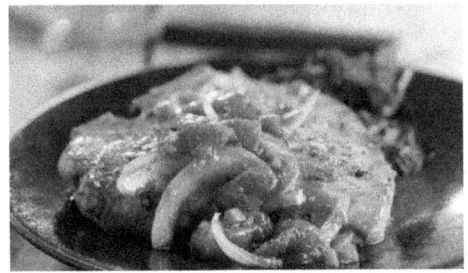

Preparation time: 15 minutes

Cooking time: 15 minutes

Servings: 2

Level of difficulty: Normal

Category: Leaner

Ingredients:

- 4 (5-ounce) bone-free pork chops, ½-inch thick and fat-cut

- 2 teaspoons of salt-free extra-spicy seasoning cubes
- ½ small yellow onion, sliced
- 1 jalapeño pepper, finely chopped and seeded
- 1 (14.5-ounce) canned diced tomatoes, undrained

Directions:

1. Using spicy seasoning mix on both sides of pork chops. Cover a large non-stick skillet with spray and heat the pan over medium to high heat.
2. Add onion and jalapeño, sautéing for around 2 minutes until slightly tender. Push the mix to one side of the skillet.
3. Add pork chops on the other side of the skillet. Cook the pork chops for 3 minutes, rotating once so that both sides are browned evenly.
4. Put tomatoes into the saucepan. When the liquid starts boiling, lower the heat to low and cover with a lid. Cook for around 6 to 8 minutes until the pork chops are no longer pink in the middle. Serve chops, spoon them over with sauce.

Nutrition:

Calories: 270

Carbs: 6g

Fat: 13g

Protein: 32g

15. Pesto Zucchini Noodles

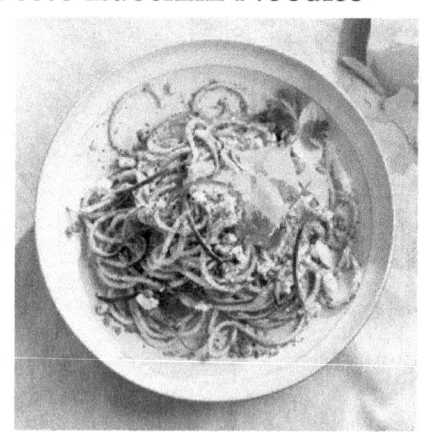

Preparation Time: 15 minutes

Cooking Time: minutes 15 minutes

Level of difficulty: Normal

Servings: 4

Category: Green

Ingredients:

- 4 zucchinis, spiralized
- 1 tbsp avocado oil
- 2 garlic cloves, chopped
- 2/3 cup olive oil
- 1/3 cup parmesan cheese, grated
- 2 cups fresh basil
- 1/3 cup almonds
- 1/8 tsp black pepper
- ¾ tsp sea salt

Directions:

1. Add zucchini noodles into a colander and sprinkle with ¼ teaspoon of salt.

Cover and let sit for 30 minutes. Drain zucchini noodles well and pat dry. Preheat the oven to 400 F.

2. Place almonds on a parchment-lined baking sheet and bake for 6-8 minutes. Transfer toasted almonds into the food processor and process until coarse.

3. Add olive oil, cheese, basil, garlic, pepper, and remaining salt in a food processor with almonds and process until pesto texture.

4. Warm your avocado oil in a large pan over medium-high heat, then put zucchini noodles and cook for 4-5 minutes.

5. Pour pesto over zucchini noodles, mix well and cook for 1 minute. Serve immediately with baked salmon.

Nutrition:

Calories: 525 Fat 44 g Carbs 3 g Protein 16 g

16. Baked Cod & Vegetables

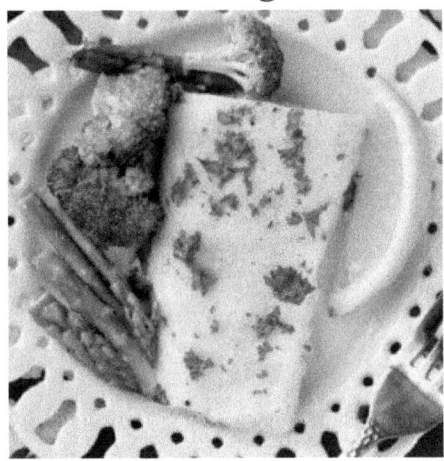

Preparation Time: 15 minutes

Cooking Time: 15 minutes

Servings: 4

Level of difficulty: Normal

Category: Green

Ingredients:

- 1 lb. cod fillets
- 8 oz asparagus, chopped
- 3 cups broccoli, chopped
- ¼ cup parsley, minced
- ½ tsp lemon pepper seasoning
- ½ tsp paprika
- ¼ cup olive oil
- ¼ cup lemon juice - 1 tsp salt

Directions:

1. Warm oven to 400 F. Line a baking sheet with parchment paper and set aside. Mix the lemon juice, paprika, olive oil, pepper spices, and salt in a small bowl.

2. Put the fish fillets in the middle of the greaseproof paper. Arrange the broccoli and asparagus around the fish fillets.

3. Pour lemon juice mixture over the fish fillets and top with parsley. Bake in preheated oven for 13-15 minutes. Serve and enjoy.

Nutrition:

Calories 240 Fat 11 g Carbs 6 g Protein 27 g

17. Parmesan Zucchini

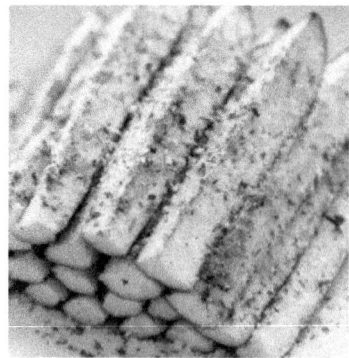

Preparation Time: 15 minutes

Cooking Time: 15 minutes

Servings: 4

Level of difficulty: Easy

Category: Green

Ingredients:

- 4 zucchinis, quartered lengthwise
- 2 tbsp fresh parsley, chopped
- 2 tbsp olive oil
- ¼ tsp garlic powder
- ½ tsp dried basil
- ½ tsp dried oregano
- ½ tsp dried thyme
- ½ cup parmesan cheese, grated
- Pepper
- Salt

Directions:

1. Warm oven to 350 F. Line baking sheet with parchment paper and set aside. Mix parmesan cheese, garlic powder, basil, oregano, thyme, pepper, and salt in a small bowl.
2. Arrange zucchini onto the prepared baking sheet and drizzle with oil and sprinkle with parmesan cheese mixture.
3. Bake in the preheated oven within 15 minutes, then broil for 2 minutes or until lightly golden brown. Garnish with parsley and serve immediately.

Nutrition:

Calories 244 Fat 14 g Carbs 7 g Protein 15 g

18. Chicken Zucchini Noodles

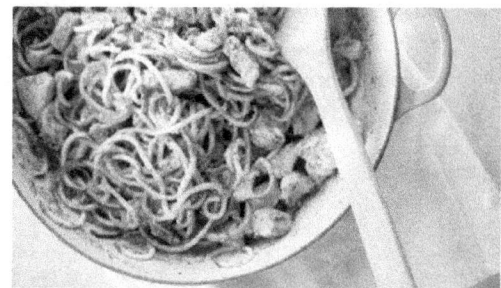

Preparation Time: 20 minutes

Cooking Time: 5 minutes

Servings: 2

Level of difficulty: Normal

Category: Leaner

Ingredients:

- 1 large zucchini, spiralized
- 1 chicken breast, skinless & boneless
- ½ tbsp jalapeno, minced

- 2 garlic cloves, minced
- ½ tsp ginger, minced
- ½ tbsp fish sauce
- 2 tbsp coconut cream
- ½ tbsp honey
- ½ lime juice
- 1 tbsp peanut butter
- 1 carrot, chopped
- 2 tbsp cashews, chopped
- ¼ cup fresh cilantro, chopped
- 1 tbsp olive oil
- Pepper
- Salt

Directions:

1. Warm-up olive oil in a pan over medium-high heat. Season chicken breast with pepper and salt. Once the oil is hot, add chicken breast into the pan and cook for 3-4 minutes per side or until cooked.
2. Remove chicken breast from pan. Shred chicken breast with a fork and set aside.
3. Mix peanut butter, jalapeno, garlic, ginger, fish sauce, coconut cream, honey, and lime juice in a small bowl. Set aside.
4. In a large mixing bowl, combine spiralized zucchini, carrots, cashews, cilantro, and shredded chicken.
5. Pour peanut butter mixture over zucchini noodles and toss to combine. Serve immediately and enjoy.

Nutrition:

Calories 353

Fat 21 g

Carbs 20.5 g

Protein 25 g

19. Tomato Cucumber Avocado Salad

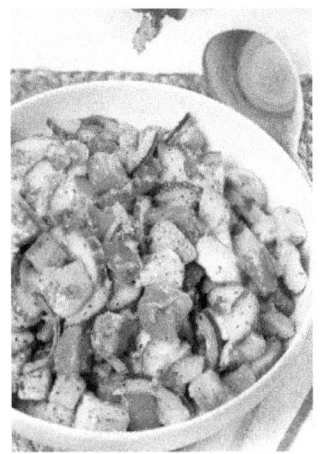

Preparation Time: 15 minutes

Cooking Time: 0 minutes

Servings: 4

Level of difficulty: Easy

Category: Green

Ingredients:

- 12 oz cherry tomatoes, cut in half
- 5 small cucumbers, chopped

- 3 small avocados, chopped
- ½ tsp ground black pepper
- 2 tbsp olive oil
- 2 tbsp fresh lemon juice
- ¼ cup fresh cilantro, chopped
- 1 tsp sea salt

Directions:

1. Add cherry tomatoes, cucumbers, avocados, and cilantro into the large mixing bowl and mix well. Mix olive oil, lemon juice, black pepper, and salt and pour over salad. Toss well and serve immediately.

Nutrition:

Calories 442 Fat 31 g Carbs 30.3 g

Protein 2 g

20. Creamy Cauliflower Soup

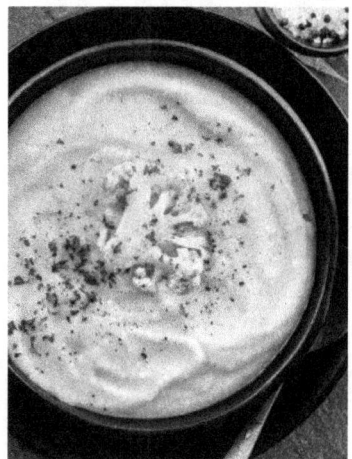

Preparation Time: 15 minutes

Cooking Time: 15 minutes

Servings: 6

Level of difficulty: Easy

Category: Green

Ingredients:

- 5 cups cauliflower rice
- 8 oz cheddar cheese, grated
- 2 cups unsweetened almond milk
- 2 cups vegetable stock
- 2 tbsp water
- 1 small onion, chopped
- 2 garlic cloves, minced
- 1 tbsp olive oil
- Pepper
- Salt

Directions:

1. Warm-up olive oil in a large stockpot over medium heat. Add onion and garlic and cook for 1-2 minutes. Add cauliflower rice and water. Cover and cook for 5-7 minutes.

2. Now add vegetable stock and almond milk and stir well. Bring to boil. Turn heat to low and simmer for 5 minutes.

3. Turn off the heat. Slowly add cheddar cheese and stir until smooth—season soup with pepper and salt. Stir well and serve hot.

Nutrition:

Calories 214 Fat 15 g Carbs 3 g Protein 16 g

21. Taco Zucchini Boats

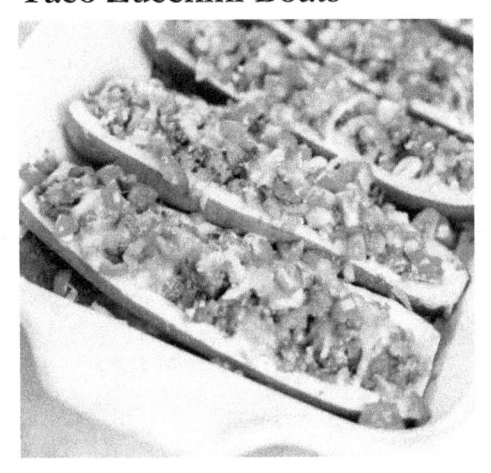

Preparation Time: 20 minutes

Cooking Time: 55 minutes

Servings: 4

Level of difficulty: Normal

Category: Lean

Ingredients:

- 4 medium zucchinis, cut in half lengthwise
- ¼ cup fresh cilantro, chopped
- ½ cup cheddar cheese, shredded
- ¼ cup of water
- 4 oz tomato sauce
- 2 tbsp bell pepper, mined
- ½ small onion, minced
- ½ tsp oregano
- 1 tsp paprika
- 1 tsp chili powder
- 1 tsp cumin
- 1 tsp garlic powder
- 1 lb. lean ground turkey
- ½ cup of salsa
- 1 tsp kosher salt

Directions:

1. Preheat the oven to 400 F. Add ¼ cup of salsa to the bottom of the baking dish. Using a spoon, hollow out the center of the zucchini halves.
2. Chop the scooped-out flesh of zucchini and set aside ¾ cup of chopped flesh. Add zucchini halves to the boiling water and cook for 1 minute. Remove zucchini halves from water.
3. Add ground turkey in a large pan and cook until meat is no longer pink. Add spices and mix well.
4. Add reserved zucchini flesh, water, tomato sauce, bell pepper, and onion. Stir well and cover, simmer over low heat for 20 minutes.
5. Stuff zucchini boats with taco meat and top each with one tablespoon of shredded cheddar cheese. Place zucchini boats in a baking dish—cover dish with foil and bake within 35 minutes.
6. Top with remaining salsa and chopped cilantro. Serve and enjoy.

Nutrition:

Calories 297 Fat 17 g Carbs 12 g Protein 30.2 g

22. Broccoli Salad

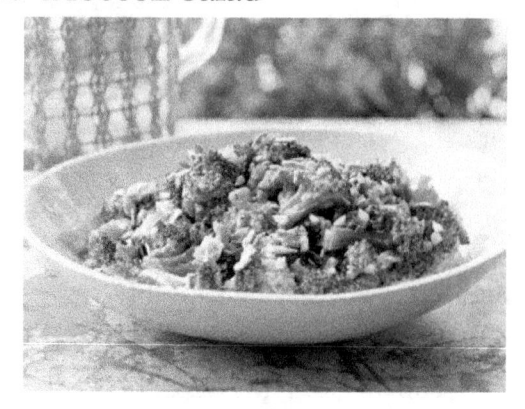

Preparation Time: 25 minutes

Cooking Time: 0 minutes

Servings: 6

Level of difficulty: Easy

Category: Green

Ingredients:

- 3 cups broccoli, chopped
- 1 tbsp apple cider vinegar
- ½ cup Greek yogurt
- 2 tbsp sunflower seeds
- 3 bacon slices, cooked and chopped
- 1/3 cup onion, sliced
- ¼ tsp stevia

Directions:

1. In a mixing bowl, mix broccoli, onion, and bacon. In a small bowl, mix yogurt, vinegar, and stevia and pour over broccoli mixture. Stir to combine.
2. Sprinkle sunflower seeds on top of the salad—store salad in the refrigerator for 30 minutes. Serve and enjoy.

Nutrition:

Calories 90 Fat 9 g Carbs 4 g Protein 2 g

23. Zucchini Quiche

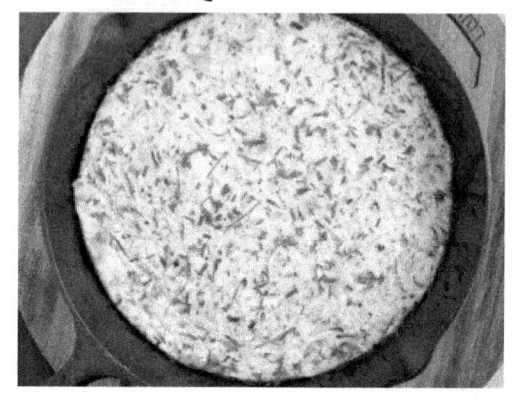

Preparation Time: 25 minutes

Cooking Time: 1 hour

Servings: 8

Level of difficulty: Normal

Category: Green

Ingredients:

- 6 eggs
- 2 medium zucchinis, shredded
- ½ tsp dried basil
- 2 garlic cloves, minced
- 1 tbsp dry onion, minced
- 2 tbsp parmesan cheese, grated

- 2 tbsp fresh parsley, chopped
- ½ cup olive oil
- 1 cup cheddar cheese, shredded
- ¼ cup coconut flour
- ¾ cup almond flour
- ½ tsp salt

Directions:

1. Warm oven to 350 F. Grease a 9-inch pie pan and set aside. Squeeze excess liquid from zucchini. Put all fixings into a large bowl and mix until well combined. Pour into the prepared cake pan.
2. Bake in a preheated oven for 45-60 minutes or until cooked through. Remove from the oven and let it cool completely. Slice and serve.

Nutrition:

Calories 288 Fat 23 g Carbs 5 g Protein 11 g

24. Turkey Spinach Egg Muffins

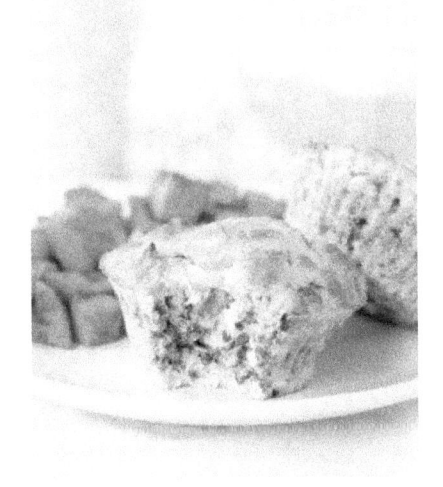

Preparation Time: 10 minutes

Cooking Time: 20 minutes

Servings: 3

Level of difficulty: Normal

Category: Leanest

Ingredients:

- 5 egg whites
- 2 eggs
- ¼ cup cheddar cheese, shredded
- ¼ cup spinach, chopped
- ¼ cup milk
- 3 lean breakfast turkey sausage
- Pepper
- Salt

Directions:

1. Warm oven to 350 F. Grease muffin tray cups and sets aside. In a pan, brown the turkey sausage links over medium-high heat until the sausage is brown from all the sides.
2. Cut sausage into ½-inch pieces and set aside. In a large bowl, whisk together eggs, egg whites, milk, pepper, and salt. Stir in spinach.
3. Pour egg mixture into the prepared muffin tray. Divide sausage and cheese evenly between each muffin cup.

4. Bake in the preheated oven within 20 minutes or until muffins are set. Serve warm and enjoy.

Nutrition:

Calories 123

Fat 8 g

Carbs 9 g

Protein 13 g

25. Chicken Casserole

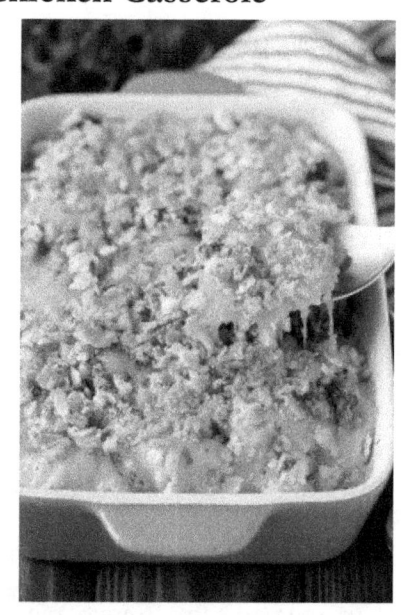

Preparation Time: 15 minutes

Cooking Time: 40 minutes

Servings: 4

Level of difficulty: Easy

Category: Leaner

Ingredients:

- 1 lb. cooked chicken, shredded
- ¼ cup Greek yogurt
- 1 cup cheddar cheese, shredded
- ½ cup of salsa
- 4 oz cream cheese, softened
- 4 cups cauliflower florets
- 1/8 tsp black pepper
- ½ tsp kosher salt

Directions:

1. Add cauliflower florets into the microwave-safe dish and cook for 10 minutes or until tender.
2. Add cream cheese and microwave for 30 seconds more. Stir well.
3. Add chicken, yogurt, cheddar cheese, salsa, pepper, and salt, and stir everything well.
4. Preheat the oven to 375 F. Bake in preheated oven for 20 minutes.
5. Serve hot and enjoy.

Nutrition:

Calories 429

Fat 23 g

Carbs 6 g

Protein 44 g

26. Aloo Gobi

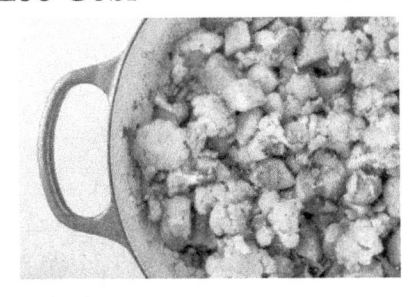

Preparation Time: 15 Minutes

Cooking time: 4 to 5 hours

Servings: 4

Level of difficulty: Normal

Category: Green

Ingredients:

- 1 large cauliflower, cut into 1-inch pieces
- 1 large russet potato, peeled and diced
- 1 medium yellow onion, peeled and diced
- 1 cup canned diced tomatoes, with juice
- 1 cup frozen peas - ¼ cup of water
- 1 fresh ginger, peeled & finely chopped
- 1½ teaspoons minced garlic (3 cloves)
- 1 jalapeño pepper, stemmed and sliced
- 1 tablespoon cumin seeds
- 1 tablespoon garam masala
- 1 teaspoon ground turmeric
- 1 heaping tablespoon fresh cilantro
- Cooked rice, for serving (optional)

Directions:

1. Combine the cauliflower, potato, onion, diced tomatoes, peas, water, ginger, garlic, jalapeño, cumin seeds, garam masala, and turmeric in a slow cooker; mix until well combined.
2. Cover and cook on low within 4 to 5 hours. Garnish with cilantro, and serve over cooked rice (if using).

Nutrition:

Calories: 115 Fat: 1g Protein: 6g Carbs: 0g

27. Jackfruit Carnitas

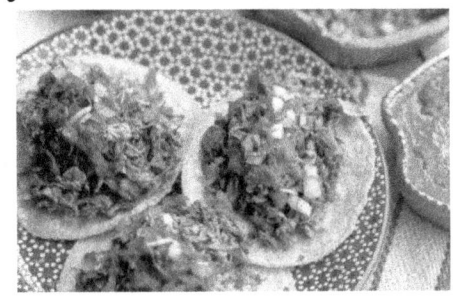

Preparation Time: 15 Minutes

Cooking Time: 8 Hours

Level of difficulty: Normal

Servings: 4

Category: Green

Ingredients:

- 2 (20-ounce) cans jackfruit, drained, hard pieces discarded

- ¾ cup vegetable broth
- 1 tablespoon ground cumin
- 1 tablespoon dried oregano
- 1½ teaspoons ground coriander
- 1 teaspoon minced garlic (2 cloves)
- ½ teaspoon ground cinnamon
- 2 bay leaves
- Tortillas, for serving
- Optional toppings: diced onions, sliced radishes, fresh cilantro, lime wedges, nacho cheese

Directions:

1. Combine the jackfruit, vegetable broth, cumin, oregano, coriander, garlic, cinnamon, and bay leaves in a slow cooker. Stir to combine.
2. Cover and cook on low within 8 hours or on high for 4 hours. Use two forks to pull the jackfruit apart into shreds. Remove the bay leaves. Serve in warmed tortillas with your favorite taco fixings.

Nutrition:

Calories: 286

Fat: 2g

Protein: 6g

Carbs: 0g

28. Baked Beans

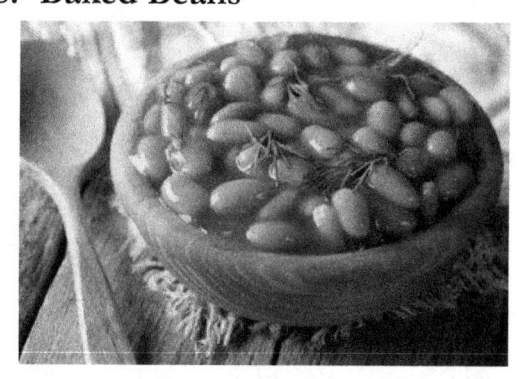

Preparation Time: 15 Minutes

Cooking Time: 6 Hours

Servings: 4

Level of difficulty: Easy

Category: Green

Ingredients:

- 2 cans white beans, drained and rinsed
- 1 (15-ounce) can tomato sauce
- 1 medium yellow onion, finely diced
- 1½ teaspoons minced garlic (3 cloves)
- 3 tablespoons brown sugar
- 2 tablespoons molasses
- 1 tablespoon prepared yellow mustard
- 1 tablespoon chili powder
- 1 teaspoon soy sauce
- Pinch salt
- Freshly ground black pepper

Directions:

1. Place the beans, tomato sauce, onion, garlic, brown sugar, molasses, mustard, chili powder, and soy sauce into a slow cooker; mix well. Cover and cook on low within 6 hours. Season with salt and pepper before serving.

Nutrition:

Calories: 468

Fat: 2g

Protein: 28g

Carbs: 30g

29. Brussels Sprouts Curry

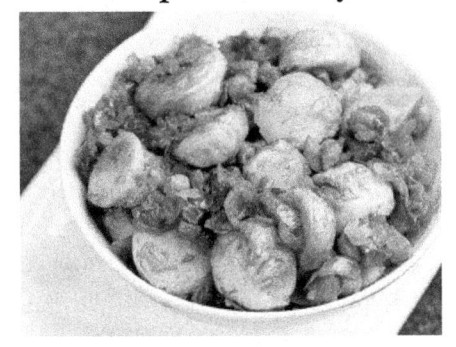

Preparation time: 15 minutes

Cooking time: 7 to 8 hours

Servings: 4

Level of difficulty: Normal

Category: Green

Ingredients:

- ¾ pound Brussels sprouts, bottoms cut off and sliced in half
- 1 can full-fat coconut milk
- 1 cup vegetable broth
- 1 medium onion, diced
- 1 medium carrot, thinly sliced
- 1 medium red or Yukon potato, diced
- 1½ teaspoons minced garlic (3 cloves)
- 1 fresh ginger, peeled & minced
- 1 small serrano chili, seeded & finely chopped
- 2 tablespoons peanut butter
- 1 tablespoon rice vinegar or other vinegar
- 1 tablespoon cane sugar or agave nectar
- 1 tablespoon soy sauce
- 1 teaspoon curry powder
- 1 teaspoon ground turmeric
- Pinch salt
- Freshly ground black pepper
- Cooked rice, for serving (optional)

Directions:

1. Place the Brussels sprouts, coconut milk, vegetable broth, onion, carrot, potato, garlic, ginger, serrano chili, peanut butter, vinegar, cane sugar, soy sauce, curry powder, and turmeric in a slow cooker. Mix well.

2. Cover and cook on low within 7 to 8 hours or on high for 4 to 5 hours—season with salt and pepper. Serve over rice (if using).

Nutrition:

Calories: 404

Fat: 29g

Protein: 10g

Carbs: 0g

30. Jambalaya

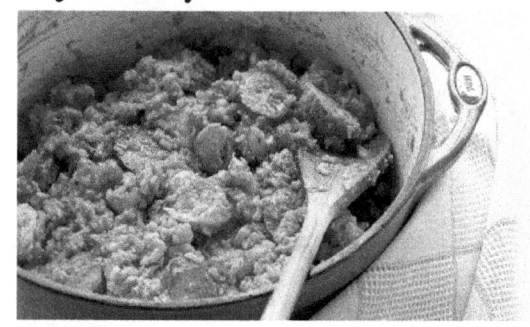

Preparation time: 15 minutes

Cooking time: 6 to 8 hours

Servings: 4

Level of difficulty: Normal

Category: Green

Ingredients:

- 2 cups vegetable broth
- 1 large yellow onion, diced
- 1 green bell pepper, seeded and chopped
- 2 celery stalks, chopped
- 1½ teaspoons minced garlic (3 cloves)
- 1 can black-eyed peas, drained and rinsed
- 1 can of (dark) red kidney beans, emptied, then rinsed
- 1 (15-ounce) can diced tomatoes, drained
- 2 tablespoons Cajun seasoning
- 2 teaspoons dried oregano
- 2 teaspoons dried parsley
- 1 teaspoon cayenne pepper
- 1 teaspoon smoked paprika
- ½ teaspoon dried thyme
- Cooked rice, for serving (optional)

Directions:

1. Combine the vegetable broth, onion, bell pepper, celery, garlic, kidney beans, black-eyed peas, diced tomatoes, Cajun seasoning, oregano, parsley, cayenne pepper, smoked paprika, and dried thyme in a slow cooker; mix well.
2. Cover and cook on low within 6 to 8 hours. Serve over rice (if using).

Nutrition:

Calories: 428

Fat: 2g

Protein: 28g

Carbs: 23g

31. Mushroom-Kale Stroganoff

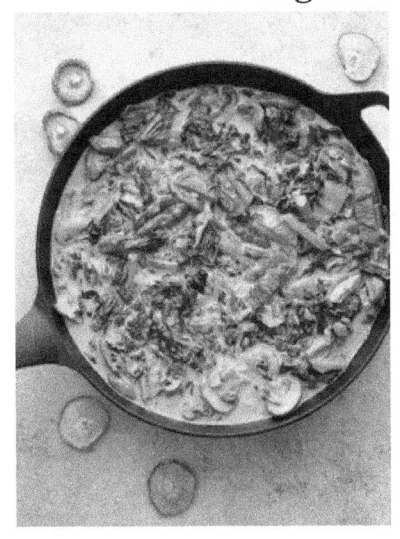

Preparation time: 15 minutes

Cooking time: 6 to 8 hours

Servings: 4

Level of difficulty: Normal

Category: Green

Ingredients:

- 1-pound mushrooms, sliced
- 1½ cups vegetable broth
- 1 cup stemmed and chopped kale
- 1 small yellow onion, diced
- 2 garlic cloves, minced
- 2 tablespoons all-purpose flour
- 2 tablespoons ketchup or tomato paste
- 2 teaspoons paprika
- ½ cup vegan sour cream
- ¼ cup chopped fresh parsley
- Cooked rice, pasta, or quinoa, for serving

Directions:

1. Combine the mushrooms, vegetable broth, kale, onion, garlic, flour, ketchup or tomato paste, and paprika in a slow cooker. Mix thoroughly.

2. Cover and cook on low within 6 to 8 hours. Stir in the sour cream and parsley just before serving. Serve over rice, pasta, or quinoa.

Nutrition:

Calories: 146 Fat: 7g Protein: 8gCarbs: 18g

32. Tomatillo and Green Chili Pork Stew

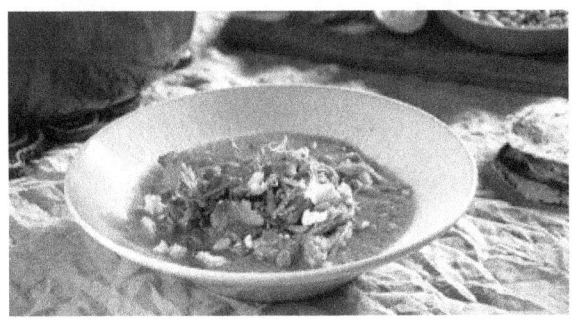

Preparation Time: 10 minutes

Cooking Time: 20 minutes

Servings: 4

Level of difficulty: Normal

Category: Green

Ingredients:

- 2 scallions, chopped

- 2 garlic cloves
- 1 lb. tomatillos, trimmed and chopped
- 8 large romaine or green lettuce leaves, divided
- 2 serrano chilies, seeds, and membranes
- ½ tsp. dried Mexican oregano (or you can use regular oregano)
- 1 ½ lb. of boneless pork loin, to be cut into bite-sized cubes
- ¼ cup cilantro, chopped
- ¼ tbsp. (each) salt and paper
- 1 jalapeño, seeds and membranes to be removed and thinly sliced
- 1 cup sliced radishes
- 4 lime wedges

Directions:

1. Combine scallions, garlic, tomatillos, 4 lettuce leaves, serrano chilies, and oregano in a blender. Then purée until smooth.
2. Put pork and tomatillo mixture in a medium pot. 1-inch of purée should cover the pork; if not, add water until it covers it. Season with pepper & salt, and cover it. Simmer on the heat for approximately 20 minutes.
3. Now, finely shred the remaining lettuce leaves. When the stew is done cooking, garnish with cilantro, radishes, finely shredded lettuce, sliced jalapeños, and lime wedges.

Nutrition:

Calories: 370

Fats: 19 g

Carbs: 14 g

Protein: 36 g

33. Avocado Lime Shrimp Salad

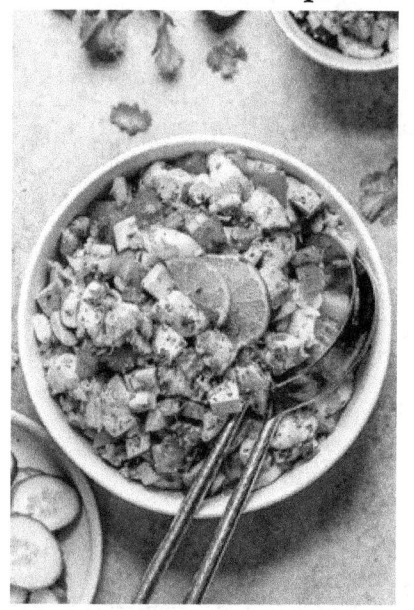

Preparation Time: 15 minutes

Cooking Time: 0 minutes

Servings: 2

Level of difficulty: Easy

Category: Leanest

Ingredients:

- 14 ounces jumbo cooked shrimp, chopped

- 4 ½ ounces avocado, diced
- 1 ½ cup tomato, diced
- ¼ cup chopped green onion
- ¼ cup jalapeño with the seeds removed, diced finely
- 1 tsp. olive oil
- 2 tbsp. lime juice
- 1/8 tsp. salt
- 1 tbsp. chopped cilantro

Directions:

1. Get a small bowl and combine green onion, olive oil, lime juice, pepper, and salt pinch. Wait for about 5 minutes for all of them to marinate and mellow the flavor of the onion.
2. Get a large bowl and combine chopped shrimp, tomato, avocado, jalapeño. Combine all of the ingredients, add cilantro, and gently toss. Add pepper and salt as desired.

Nutrition:

Calories: 314

Carbs: 15 g

Fiber: 9 g

Protein: 26 g

34. Grilled Mahi-Mahi with Jicama Slaw

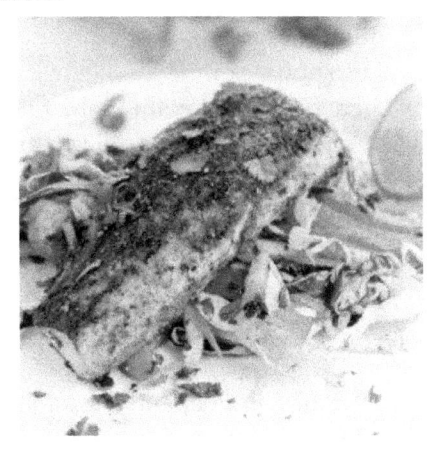

Preparation Time: 20 minutes

Cooking Time: 10 minutes

Servings: 4

Level of difficulty: Normal

Category: Leanest

Ingredients:

- 1 tsp. each for pepper and salt, divided
- 1 tbsp. lime juice, divided
- 2 tbsp. + 2 teaspoons of extra virgin olive oil
- 4 raw mahi-mahi fillets, which should be about 8 oz. each
- ½ cucumber, thinly cut into long strips
- 1 jicama, thinly slice into long strips
- 1 cup alfalfa sprouts
- 2 cups coarsely chopped watercress

Directions:

1. Combine ½ teaspoon of both pepper and salt, 1 teaspoon of lime juice, and 2 teaspoons of oil in a small bowl. Then brush the mahi-mahi fillets all through with the olive oil mixture.
2. Grill the mahi-mahi on medium-high heat until it becomes done in about 5 minutes, turn it to the other side, and let it be done for about 5 minutes.
3. For the slaw, combine the watercress, cucumber, jicama, and alfalfa sprouts in a bowl. Now combine ½ teaspoon of both pepper and salt, 2 teaspoons of lime juice, and 2 tablespoons of extra virgin oil in a small bowl. Drizzle it over slaw and toss together to combine.

Nutrition:

Calories: 320

Fat: 11 g

Carbs: 10 g

Protein: 44 g

35. Rosemary Cauliflower Rolls

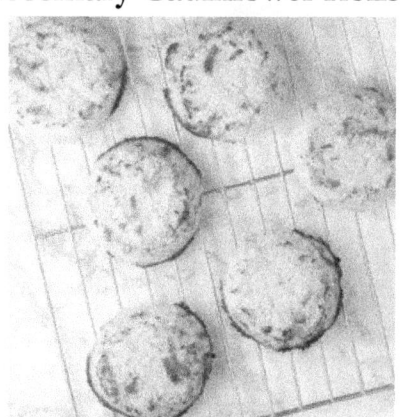

Preparation Time: 10 minutes

Cooking Time: 30 minutes

Servings: 3

Level of difficulty: Normal

Category: Green

Ingredients:

- 1/3 cup almond flour
- 4 cups riced cauliflower
- 1/3 cup reduced-fat, shredded mozzarella or cheddar cheese
- 2 eggs
- 2 tbsp. fresh rosemary, finely chopped
- ½ tsp. salt

Directions:

1. Preheat your oven to 400°F. Combine all the listed ingredients in a medium-sized bowl.
2. Scoop cauliflower mixture into 12 evenly-sized rolls/biscuits onto a lightly-greased and foil-lined baking sheet. Bake until it turns golden brown, which should be achieved in about 30 minutes.

Nutrition:

Calories: 254Fats: 8 g

Carbs: 7 g Protein: 24 g

CHAPTER 5:

Breakfast

36. Alkaline Blueberry Spelt Pancakes

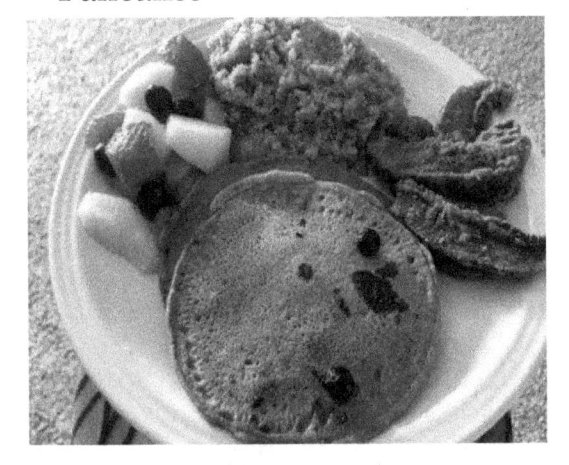

Preparation Time: 6 minutes

Cooking Time: 20 minutes

Servings: 3

Level of difficulty: Easy

Category: Green

Ingredients:

- 2 cups spelt flour
- 1 cup of coconut milk
- 1/2 cup alkaline water
- 2 tbsps. grapeseed oil
- 1/2 cup agave
- 1/2 cup blueberries
- 1/4 tsp. sea moss

Directions:

1. Mix the spelt flour, agave, grapeseed oil, hemp seeds, and sea moss in a bowl. Add in 1 cup of hemp milk and alkaline water to the mixture until you get the consistency mixture you like.

2. Crimp the blueberries into the batter. Heat the skillet to moderate heat, then lightly coat it with the grapeseed oil.

3. Pour the batter into the skillet, then let them cook for approximately 5 minutes on every side. Serve and Enjoy.

Nutrition:

Calories: 203

Fat: 1.4g

Carbs: 41.6g

Proteins: 4.8g

37. Alkaline Blueberry Muffins

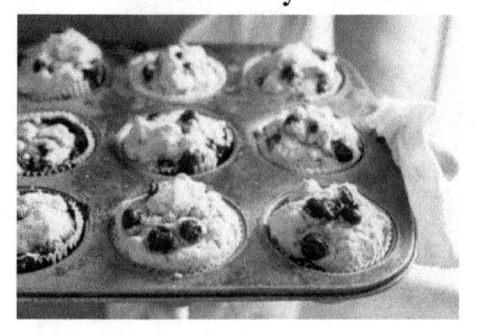

Preparation Time: 5 Minutes

Cooking Time: 20 minutes

Servings: 3

Level of difficulty: Easy

Category: Green

Ingredients:

- 1 cup of coconut milk
- 3/4 cup spelt flour
- 3/4 teff flour
- 1/2 cup blueberries
- 1/3 cup agave
- 1/4 cup sea moss gel
- 1/2 tsp. sea salt
- grapeseed oil

Directions:

1. Adjust the temperature of the oven to 365 degrees. Grease 6 regular-size muffin cups with muffin liners.
2. In a bowl, mix sea salt, sea moss, agave, coconut milk, and flour gel until they are properly blended. You then crimp in blueberries.
3. Coat the muffin pan lightly with the grapeseed oil. Pour in the muffin batter. Bake for at least 30 minutes until it turns golden brown. Serve.

Nutrition:

Calories: 160 Fat: 5g

Carbs: 25g Proteins: 2g

38. Crunchy Quinoa Meal

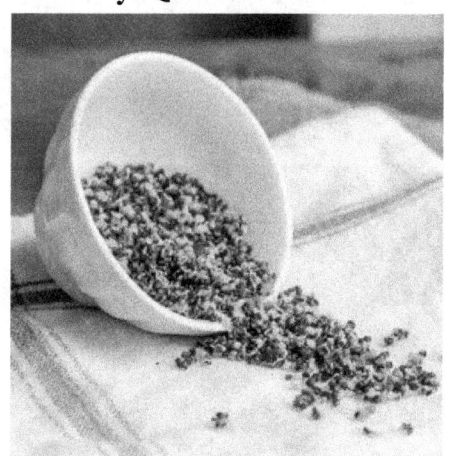

Preparation Time: 5 minutes

Cooking Time: 25 minutes

Servings: 2

Level of difficulty: Easy

Category: Healthy Fat

Ingredients:

- 3 cups of coconut milk
- 1 cup rinsed quinoa
- 1/8 tsp. ground cinnamon

- 1 cup raspberry
- 1/2 cup chopped coconuts

Directions:

1. In a saucepan, pour milk and bring to a boil over moderate heat. Add the quinoa to the milk, and then bring it to a boil once more.
2. You then let it simmer for at least 15 minutes on medium heat until the milk is reduced. Stir in the cinnamon, then mix properly.
3. Cover it, then cook for 8 minutes until the milk is completely absorbed. Add the raspberry and cook the meal for 30 seconds. Serve and enjoy.

Nutrition:

Calories: 271 Fat: 3.7g Carbs: 54g

Proteins: 6.5g

39. Coconut Pancakes

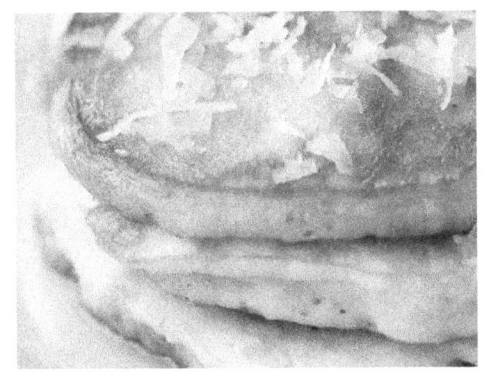

Preparation Time: 5 minutes

Cooking Time: 15 minutes

Servings: 4

Level of difficulty: Easy

Category: Healthy Fat

Ingredients:

- 1 cup coconut flour
- 2 tbsps. arrowroot powder
- 1 tsp. baking powder
- 1 cup of coconut milk
- 3 tbsps. coconut oil

Directions:

1. In a medium container, mix in all the dry ingredients. Add the coconut milk and 2 tbsp of the coconut oil, then mix properly.
2. In a skillet, dissolve 1 tsp of coconut oil. Put the batter into the skillet, then swirl the pan to spread the batter evenly into a smooth pancake.
3. Cook it for like 3 minutes on medium heat until it becomes firm. Turn the pancake to the other side, then cook it for another 2 minutes until it turns golden brown.
4. Cook the remaining pancakes in the same process. Serve.

Nutrition:

Calories: 377

Fat: 14.9g

Carbs: 60.7g

Protein: 6.4g

40. Quinoa Porridge

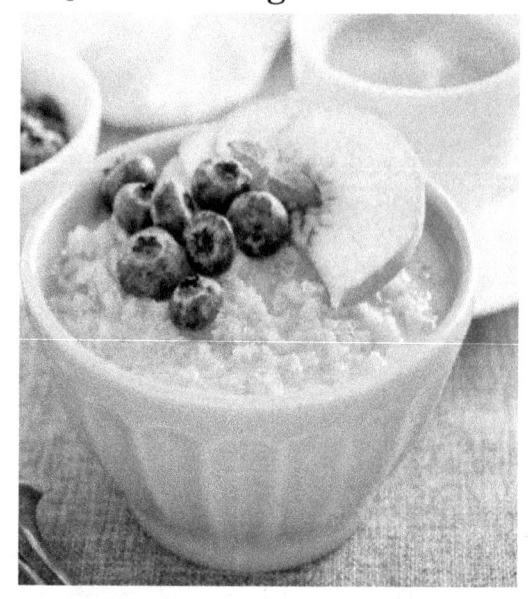

Preparation Time: 5 minutes

Cooking Time: 25 minutes

Servings: 2

Level of difficulty: Easy

Category: Green

Ingredients:

- 2 cups of coconut milk
- 1 cup rinsed quinoa
- 1/8 tsp. ground cinnamon
- 1 cup fresh blueberries

Directions:

1. In a saucepan, boil the coconut milk over high heat. Add the quinoa to the milk, then bring the mixture to a boil.
2. You then let it simmer for 15 minutes on medium heat until the milk is reducing. Add the cinnamon, then mix it properly in the saucepan.
3. Cover the saucepan and cook for at least 8 minutes until the milk is completely absorbed. Add in the blueberries, then cook for 30 more seconds. Serve.

Nutrition:

Calories: 271

Fat: 3.7g

Carbs: 54g

Protein: 6.5g

41. Amaranth Porridge

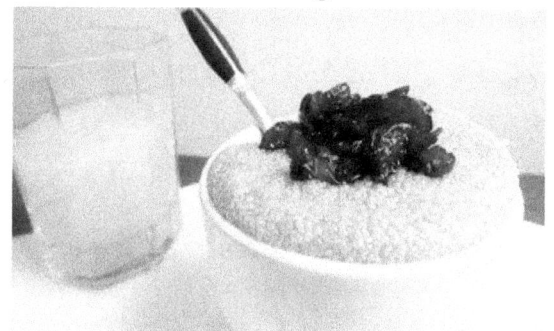

Preparation Time: 5 minutes

Cooking Time: 30 minutes

Servings: 2

Level of difficulty: Easy

Category: Green

Ingredients:

- 2 cups of coconut milk
- 2 cups alkaline water

- 1 cup amaranth
- 2 tbsps. coconut oil
- 1 tbsp. ground cinnamon

Directions:

1. In a saucepan, mix the milk with water, then boil the mixture. You stir in the amaranth, then reduce the heat to medium.
2. Cook on medium heat then simmers for at least 30 minutes as you stir it occasionally. Turn off the heat. Add in cinnamon and coconut oil, then stir. Serve.

Nutrition:

Calories: 434 Fat: 35g

Carbs: 27g Protein: 6.7g

42. Banana Barley Porridge

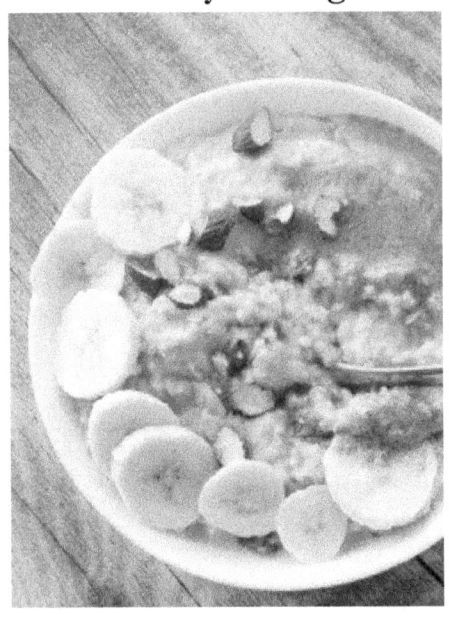

Preparation Time: 15 minutes

Cooking Time: 5 minutes

Servings: 2

Level of difficulty: Easy

Category: Healthy Fat

Ingredients:

- 1 cup divided unsweetened coconut milk
- 1 small peeled and sliced banana
- 1/2 cup barley
- 3 drops liquid stevia
- 1/4 cup chopped coconuts

Directions:

1. In a bowl, properly mix barley with half of the coconut milk and stevia. Cover the mixing bowl, then refrigerate for about 6 hours.
2. In a saucepan, mix the barley mixture with coconut milk—Cook for about 5 minutes on moderate heat. Then top it with the chopped coconuts and the banana slices. Serve.

Nutrition:

Calories: 159

Fat: 8.4g

Carbs: 19.8g

Proteins: 4.6g

43. Zucchini Muffins

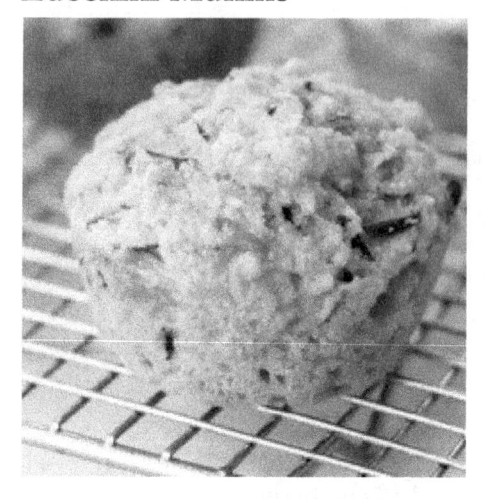

Preparation Time: 10 minutes

Cooking Time: 25 minutes

Servings: 16

Level of difficulty: Easy

Category: Green

Ingredients:

- 1 tbsp. ground flaxseed
- 3 tbsps. alkaline water
- 1/4 cup walnut butter
- 3 medium over-ripe bananas
- 2 small grated zucchinis
- 1/2 cup coconut milk
- 1 tsp. vanilla extract
- 2 cups coconut flour
- 1 tbsp. baking powder
- 1 tsp. cinnamon
- 1/4 tsp. sea salt

Directions:

1. Tune the temperature of your oven to 375°F. Grease the muffin tray with the cooking spray.
2. In a bowl, mix the flaxseed with water. In a glass bowl, mash the bananas, then stir in the remaining ingredients.
3. Properly mix and then divide the mixture into the muffin tray. Bake it for 25 minutes. Serve.

Nutrition:

Calories: 127 Fat: 6.6g Carbs: 13g

Protein: 0.7g

44. Millet Porridge

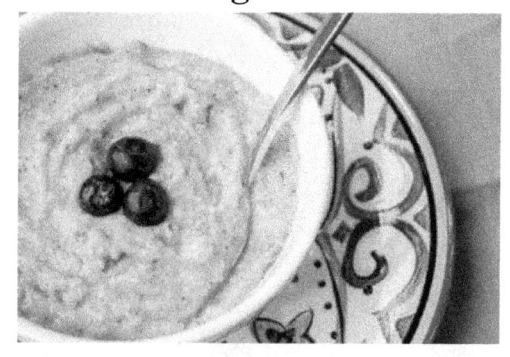

Preparation Time: 10 minutes

Cooking Time: 20 minutes

Servings: 2

Level of difficulty: Easy

Category: Green

Ingredients:

- Sea salt

- 1 tbsp. finely chopped coconuts
- 1/2 cup unsweetened coconut milk
- 1/2 cup rinsed and drained millet
- 1-1/2 cups alkaline water
- 3 drops liquid stevia

Directions:

1. Sauté the millet in a non-stick skillet for about 3 minutes. Add salt and water, then stir. Let the meal boil, then reduce the amount of heat.
2. Cook for 15 minutes, then add the remaining ingredients. Stir—Cook the meal for 4 extra minutes. Serve the meal with a topping of the chopped nuts.

Nutrition:

Calories: 219 Fat: 4.5g

Carbs: 38.2g Protein: 6.4g

45. Jackfruit Vegetable Fry

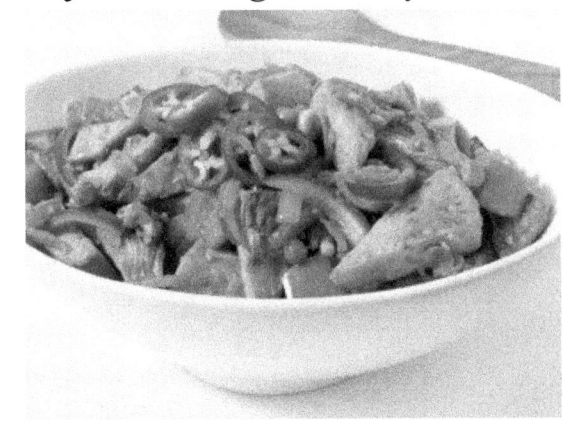

Preparation Time: 5 minutes

Cooking Time: 5 minutes

Servings: 6

Level of difficulty: Easy

Category: Green

Ingredients:

- 2 finely chopped small onions
- 2 cups finely chopped cherry tomatoes
- 1/8 tsp. ground turmeric
- 1 tbsp. olive oil
- 2 seeded and chopped red bell peppers
- 3 cups seeded and chopped firm jackfruit
- 1/8 tsp. cayenne pepper
- 2 tbsps. chopped fresh basil leaves
- Salt

Directions:

1. In a greased skillet, sauté the onions and bell peppers for about 5 minutes. Add the tomatoes, then stir. Cook for 2 minutes.
2. Then add the jackfruit, cayenne pepper, salt, and turmeric—Cook for about 8 minutes. Garnish the meal with basil leaves. Serve warm.

Nutrition:

Calories: 236 Fat: 1.8g

Carbs: 48.3g Protein: 7g

46. Zucchini Pancakes

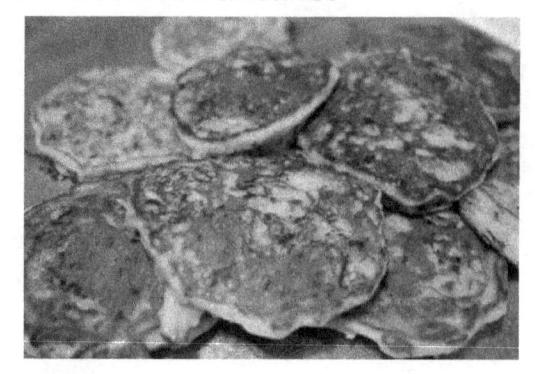

Preparation Time: 15 minutes

Cooking Time: 8 minutes

Servings: 8

Level of difficulty: Easy

Category: Green

Ingredients:

- 12 tbsps. alkaline water
- 6 large grated zucchinis
- Sea salt
- 4 tbsps. ground Flax Seeds
- 2 tsp. olive oil
- 2 finely chopped jalapeño peppers
- 1/2 cup finely chopped scallions

Directions:

1. In a bowl, mix water, and the flax seeds then set it aside. Pour oil into a large non-stick skillet, then heat it on medium heat. Then add the black pepper, salt, and zucchini.
2. Cook for 3 minutes, then transfer the zucchini into a large bowl. Add the flaxseed and the scallion mixture, then mix it.
3. Preheat a griddle, then grease it lightly with the cooking spray. Pour 1/4 of the zucchini mixture into the griddle, then cook for 3 minutes.
4. Flip the side carefully, then cook for 2 more minutes. Repeat the procedure with the remaining mixture in batches. Serve.

Nutrition:

Calories: 71 Fat: 2.8g Carbs: 9.8g

Protein: 3.7g

47. Squash Hash

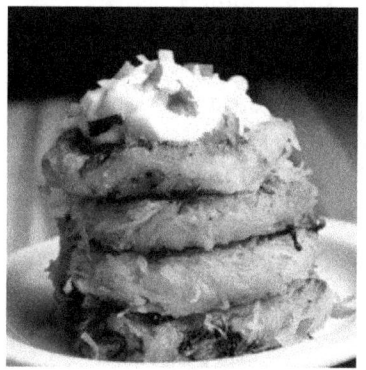

Preparation Time: 2 minutes

Cooking Time: 10 minutes

Servings: 2

Level of difficulty: Easy

Category: Green

Ingredients:

- 1 tsp. onion powder
- 1/2 cup finely chopped onion

- 2 cups spaghetti squash
- 1/2 tsp. sea salt

Directions:

1. Using paper towels, squeeze extra moisture from spaghetti squash. Place the squash into a bowl, then add the salt, onion, and the onion powder.
2. Stir properly to mix them. Spray a non-stick cooking skillet with cooking spray, then place it over moderate heat. Add the spaghetti squash to the pan.
3. Cook the squash for about 5 minutes. Flip the hash browns using a spatula. Cook for 5 minutes until the desired crispness is reached. Serve.

Nutrition: Calories: 44 Fat: 0.6g

Carbs: 9.7g Protein: 0.9g

48. Hemp Seed Porridge

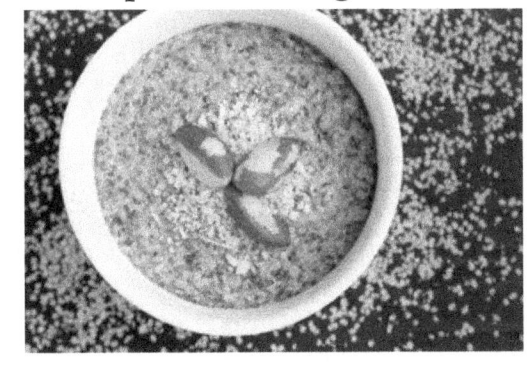

Preparation Time: 5 minutes

Cooking Time: 5 minutes

Servings: 6

Level of difficulty: Easy

Category: Green

Ingredients:

- 3 cups cooked hemp seed
- 1 packet Stevia
- 1 cup of coconut milk

Directions:

1. In a saucepan, mix the rice and the coconut milk over moderate heat for about 5 minutes as you stir it continuously. Remove the pan from the burner, then add the stevia. Stir. Serve in 6 bowls. Enjoy.

Nutrition: Protein: 7g

Calories: 236 Fat: 1.8g Carbs: 48.3g

49. Pumpkin Spice Quinoa

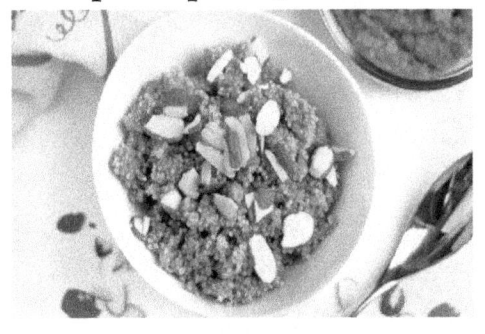

Preparation Time: 10 minutes

Cooking Time: 0 minutes

Servings: 2

Level of difficulty: Easy

Category: Green

Ingredients:

- 1 cup cooked quinoa

- 1 cup unsweetened coconut milk
- 1 large mashed banana
- 1/4 cup pumpkin puree
- 1 tsp. pumpkin spice
- 2 tsp. chia seeds

Directions:

1. In a container, mix all the ingredients. Seal the lid, then shake the container properly to mix. Refrigerate overnight. Serve.

Nutrition:

Calories: 212

Fat: 11.9g

Carbs: 31.7g

Protein: 7.3g

50. Chocolate Cherry Crunch Granola

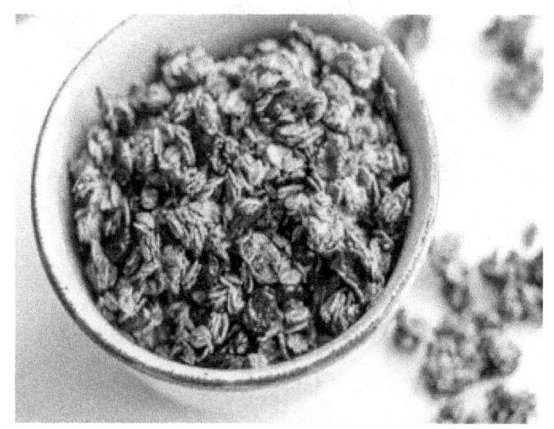

Preparation Time: 10 minutes

Cooking Time: 20 minutes

Servings: 6

Level of difficulty: Normal

Category: Healthy Fat

Ingredients:

- 3 cups rolled oats
- 2 cups assorted seeds, such as sesame, chia, sunflower, and pepitas (hulled pumpkin seeds)
- 1 cup sliced almonds
- 1 cup unsweetened coconut flakes
- 2 teaspoons vanilla extract
- 2 teaspoons ground cinnamon
- 1 teaspoon fine sea salt
- ½ cup of cocoa powder
- ½ cup pure maple syrup
- ¼ cup coconut oil or canola oil
- 1 cup dried cherries (unsweetened, if possible)
- 1 cup of chocolate chips

Directions:

1. Warm oven to 350 F. Spread 2 large baking sheets with parchment paper.
2. Stir the oats, seeds, almonds, and coconut in a large bowl. Add the vanilla, cinnamon, salt, and cocoa powder. Stir to combine.
3. In a frying pan on low, heat the maple syrup and coconut oil. Pour the warm syrup and oil over the oat

mixture and stir to coat. On the prepared baking sheets, spread the granola in even layers.

4. Bake for 15 to 18 minutes, scraping and mixing occasionally, then remove from the oven.

5. Put in the dried cherries and chocolate chips, then return to the oven, now turned off but still warm, and let the granola cool and dry thoroughly.

Nutrition:

Calories: 570

Fat: 31g

Protein: 12g

51. Mango Coconut Oatmeal

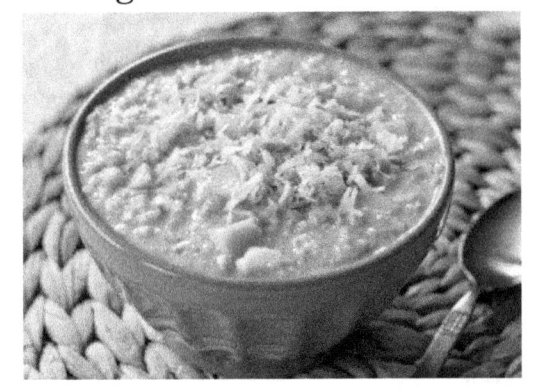

Preparation Time: 5 minutes

Cooking Time: 5 minutes

Servings: 2

Category: Green

Level of difficulty: Easy

Ingredients:

- 1½ cups water
- ½ cup 5-minute steel cut oats
- ¼ cup unsweetened canned coconut milk, plus more for serving (optional)
- 1 tablespoon pure maple syrup
- 1 teaspoon sesame seeds
- Dash ground cinnamon
- 1 mango, stripped, pitted, and divide into slices
- 1 tablespoon unsweetened coconut flakes

Directions:

1. In a frying pan over high heat, boil water. Put the oats and lower the heat. Cook, occasionally stirring, for 5 minutes.

2. Put in the coconut milk, maple syrup, and salt to combine. Get two bowls and sprinkle with the sesame seeds and cinnamon. Top with sliced mango and coconut flakes.

Nutrition:

Calories: 373

Fat: 11g

Carbs: 0g

Protein: 12g

52. Scrambled Eggs with Soy Sauce and Broccoli Slaw

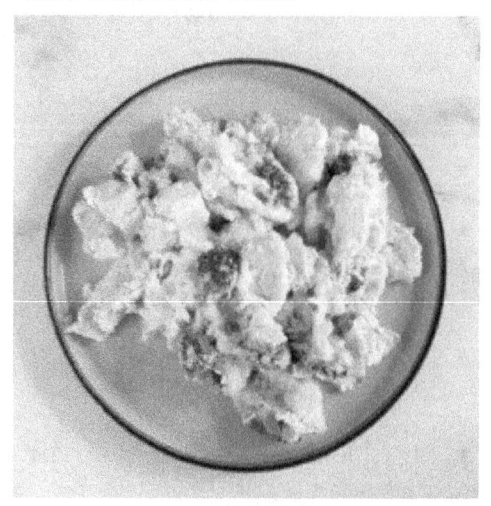

Preparation Time: 5 minutes

Cooking Time: 10 minutes

Servings: 2

Level of difficulty: Easy

Category: Green

Ingredients:

- 1 tablespoon peanut oil, divided
- 4 large eggs
- ½ to 1 tablespoon soy sauce, tamari, or Bragg's liquid aminos
- 1 tablespoon water
- 1 cup shredded broccoli slaw or other shredded vegetables
- Kosher salt
- Chopped fresh cilantro for serving
- Hot sauce, for serving

Directions:

1. In a medium non-stick skillet or cast-iron skillet over medium heat, heat 2 teaspoons of peanut oil, swirling to coat the skillet.
2. In a small bowl, whip the eggs, soy sauce, and water until smooth. Pour the eggs into the pan and let the bottom set.
3. Using a wooden spoon, spread the eggs from one side to the other a couple of times so the uncooked portions on top pool into the bottom. Cook until the eggs are set.
4. In a medium container, stir together the broccoli slaw, the remaining 1 teaspoon of peanut oil, and a touch of salt. Divide the slaw between 2 plates.
5. Top with the eggs and scatter cilantro on each serving. Serve with hot sauce.

Nutrition:

Calories: 222

Fat: 4g

Carbs: 2g

Protein: 12g

53. Tasty Breakfast Donuts

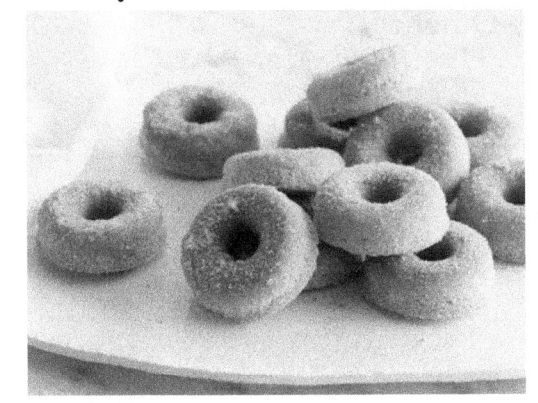

Preparation Time: 5 minutes

Cooking Time: 5 minutes

Servings: 4

Level of difficulty: Easy

Category: Healthy Fat

Ingredients:

- 43 grams' cream cheese
- 2 eggs
- 2 tablespoons almond flour
- 2 tablespoons erythritol
- 1 ½ tablespoons coconut flour
- ½ teaspoon baking powder
- ½ teaspoon vanilla extract
- 5 drops stevia (liquid form)
- 2 strips bacon, fried until crispy

Directions:

1. Rub coconut oil over donut maker and turn on. Pulse all ingredients except bacon in a blender or food processor until smooth (should take around 1 minute).
2. Pour batter into donut maker, leaving 1/10 in each round for rising. Leave for 3 minutes before flipping each donut.
3. Leave for another 2 minutes or until the fork comes out clean when piercing them. Take donuts out and let cool. Crumble bacon into bits and use to top donuts.

Nutrition: Calories: 60 Fat: 5g

Carbs: 1g Protein: 3g

54. Cheesy Spicy Bacon Bowls

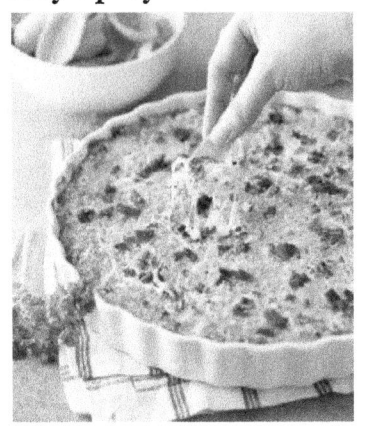

Preparation Time: 10 minutes

Cooking Time: 22 minutes

Servings: 12

Level of difficulty: Easy

Category: Lean

Ingredients:

- 6 strips bacon, pan-fried until cooked but still malleable

- 4 eggs
- 60 grams' cheddar cheese
- 40 grams' cream cheese, grated
- 2 Jalapenos, sliced and seeds removed
- 2 tablespoons coconut oil
- ¼ teaspoon onion powder
- ¼ teaspoon garlic powder
- Dash of salt and pepper

Directions:

1. Preheat oven to 375 degrees Fahrenheit.
2. In a bowl, beat together eggs, cream cheese, jalapenos (minus 6 slices), coconut oil, onion powder, garlic powder, and salt and pepper.
3. Use the leftover bacon to grease on a muffin tray, rubbing it into each insert. Place bacon wrapped inside the parameters of each insert.
4. Pour beaten mixture halfway up each bacon bowl. Garnish each bacon bowl with cheese and leftover jalapeno slices (placing one on top of each).
5. Leave in the oven for about 22 minutes, or until the egg is thoroughly cooked and cheese is bubbly. Remove from oven and let cool until edible. Enjoy!

Nutrition: Calories: 259 Fat: 24g

Carbs: 1g Protein: 10g

55. Goat Cheese Zucchini Kale Quiche

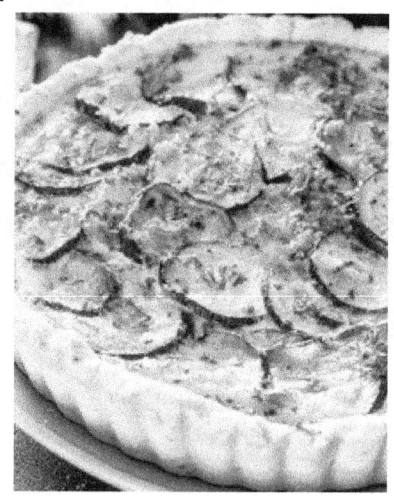

Preparation Time: 35 minutes

Cooking Time: 1 hour 10 minutes

Servings: 4

Level of difficulty: Normal

Category: Green

Ingredients:

- 4 large eggs
- 8 ounces' fresh zucchini, sliced
- 10 ounces' kale
- 3 garlic cloves (minced)
- 1 cup of soy milk
- 1 ounce's goat cheese
- 1cup grated parmesan
- 1cup shredded cheddar cheese
- 2 teaspoons olive oil
- Salt & pepper, to taste

Directions:

1. Preheat oven to 350°F. Heat-up 1 tsp of olive oil in a saucepan over medium-high heat. Sauté garlic for 1 minute until flavored.
2. Add the zucchini and cook for another 5-7 minutes until soft. Beat the eggs, and then add a little milk and Parmesan cheese.
3. Meanwhile, heat the remaining olive oil in another saucepan and add the cabbage. Cover and cook for 5 minutes until dry.
4. Slightly grease a baking dish with cooking spray and spread the kale leaves across the bottom. Add the zucchini and top with goat cheese.
5. Pour the egg, milk, and parmesan mixture evenly over the other ingredients. Top with cheddar cheese.
6. Bake for 50–60 minutes until golden brown. Check the center of the quiche; it should have a solid consistency. Let chill for a few minutes before serving.

Nutrition:

Calories: 290

Carbohydrates: 15g

Protein: 19g

Fat: 18g

56. Ricotta Ramekins

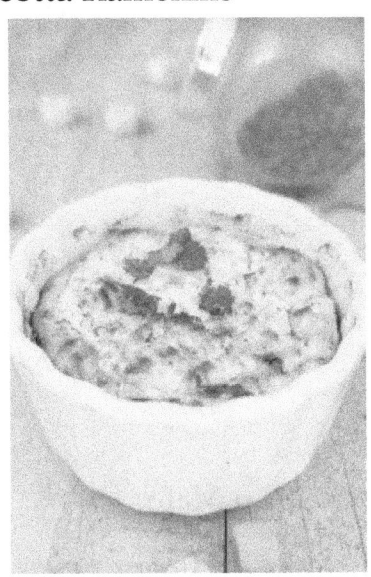

Preparation Time: 10 minutes

Cooking Time: 1 hour

Servings: 4

Level of difficulty: Easy

Category: Healthy Fat

Ingredients:

- 6 eggs, whisked
- 1 and ½ pounds ricotta cheese, soft
- ½ pound stevia
- 1 teaspoon vanilla extract
- ½ teaspoon baking powder
- Cooking spray

Directions:

1. In a bowl, mix the eggs, ricotta, and the other ingredients except for the cooking spray and whisk well.

2. Grease 4 ramekins with the cooking spray, pour the ricotta cream in each and bake at 360 degrees F for 1 hour. Serve cold.

Nutrition:

Calories 180

Fat 5.3g

Carbs 11.5g

Protein 4g

57. Chicken Lo Mein

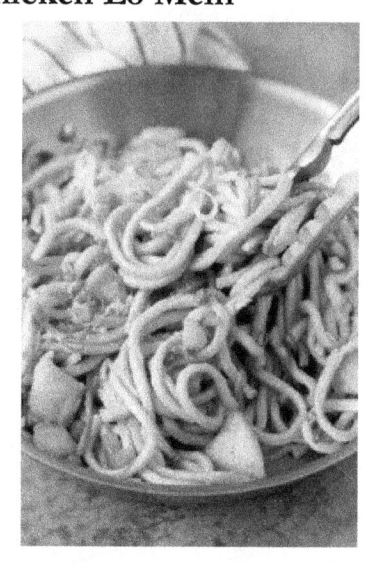

Preparation Time: 15 minutes

Cooking Time: 30 minutes

Servings: 4

Level of difficulty: Normal

Category: Leaner

Ingredients:

- 2 tbsp. + 2 tsp sesame oil, divided
- 790g boneless. skinless chicken breasts, sliced
- ¼ tsp ground black pepper
- 2 tbsp. soy sauce
- 2 tbsp. oyster sauce
- 1 garlic clove, minced
- 2 tsp peeled and minced fresh ginger-root
- 2 spring onions, trimmed and sliced with white and green parts separated
- 110 g fresh mushrooms, divided
- 1 medium red bell pepper, membranes, and seeds removed
- 2 medium zucchinis (400g), cut, sliced

Directions:

1. In a skillet, heat one teaspoon sesame oil over medium-high heat. Put the sliced chicken, season with black pepper, and cook until the chicken is done (internal temperature about 165°F). Dismiss from wok or skillet and set aside.

2. While the chicken cooks, prepare the sauce by combining the oyster sauce, soy sauce, and 2 tablespoons of sesame oil in a bowl and whisking together. Set aside.

3. With the same skillet used to cook the chicken, heat 1 teaspoon sesame oil and put the garlic, ginger, and white spring onion pieces; cook until fragrant, about 1 minute.

4. Put the mushrooms and bell peppers and continue to cook until just tender, about 3 minutes. Add zucchini noodles and toss to combine.
5. Pour in the sauce and put the chicken; cook until zucchini is tender and the mixture is heated for 5 minutes. Garnish with green parts of spring onions.

Nutrition:

Calories: 312

Protein: 9g

Fat: 10g

Carbs: 22g

58. Pancakes with Berries

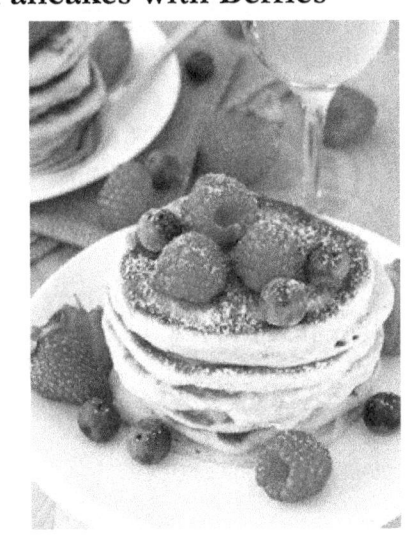

Preparation Time: 5 minutes

Cooking Time: 20 minutes

Servings: 2

Level of difficulty: Normal

Ingredients:

Category: Green

Pancake:

- 1 egg
- 50 g spelled flour
- 50 g almond flour
- 15 g coconut flour
- 150 ml of water
- salt

Filling:

- 40 g mixed berries
- 10 g chocolate
- 5 g powdered sugar
- 4 tbsp. yogurt

Directions:

1. Put the flour, egg, and some salt in a blender jar. Add 150 ml of water. Mix everything with a whisk. Heat a coated pan.
2. Put in half of the batter. Once the pancake is firm, turn it over. Take out the pancake, add the second half of the batter to the pan, and repeat.
3. Melt chocolate over a water bath. Let the pancakes cool. Brush the pancakes with the yogurt. Wash the berry and let it drain. Put berries on the yogurt.
4. Roll up the pancakes, then sprinkle them with powdered sugar. Decorate

the whole thing with the melted chocolate.

Nutrition:

Calories: 298

Carbohydrates: 26 g

Protein: 21 g

Fat: 9 g

59. Omelet À La Margherita

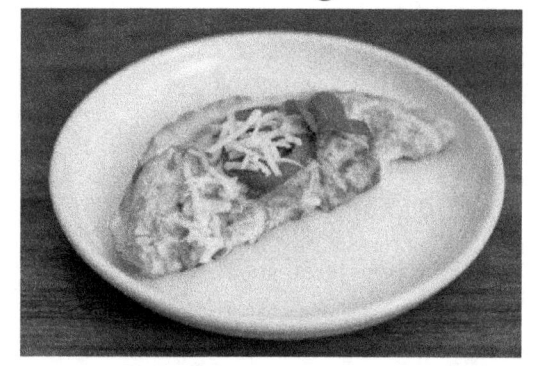

Preparation Time: 10 minutes

Cooking Time: 20 minutes

Servings: 2

Level of difficulty: Normal

Category: Lean

Ingredients:

- 3 eggs
- 50 g parmesan cheese
- 2 tbsp. heavy cream
- 1 tbsp. olive oil
- 1 teaspoon oregano
- nutmeg
- salt
- pepper

For covering:

- 3 - 4 stalks of basil
- 1 tomato
- 100 g grated mozzarella

Directions:

1. Mix the cream plus eggs in a medium bowl. Add the grated parmesan, nutmeg, oregano, pepper, and salt and stir everything. Heat the oil in a pan.

2. Add 1/2 of the egg and cream to the pan. Let the omelet set over medium heat, turn it, and then remove it.

3. Repeat with the second half of the egg mixture. Cut the tomatoes into slices and place them on top of the omelets. Scatter the mozzarella over the tomatoes.

4. Place the omelets on a baking sheet—Cook at 180 degrees for 5 to 10 minutes. Then take the omelets out and decorate them with the basil leaves.

Nutrition:

Calories: 402

Carbohydrates: 7 g

Protein: 21 g

Fat: 34 g

60. Omelet with Tomatoes and Spring Onions

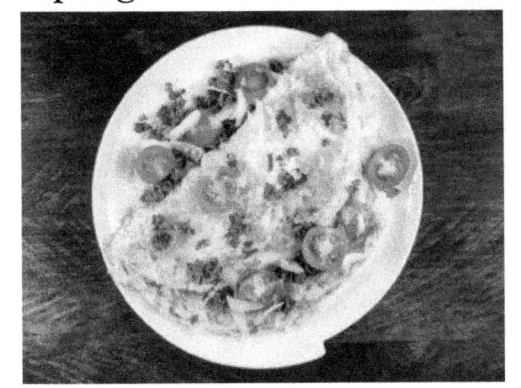

Preparation Time: 5 minutes

Cooking Time: 20 minutes

Servings: 3

Level of difficulty: Normal

Category: Green

Ingredients:

- 6 eggs - 2 tomatoes
- 2 spring onions
- 1 shallot - 2 tbsp. butter
- 1 tbsp. olive oil
- 1 pinch of nutmeg
- salt - pepper

Directions:

1. Whisk the eggs in a bowl. Mix them and season them with salt and pepper. Peel the shallot and chop it up.
2. Clean the onions and cut them into rings. Wash the tomatoes and cut them into pieces—heat butter and oil in a pan.
3. Braise half of the shallots in it, then add half the egg mixture. Let everything set over medium heat. Scatter a few tomatoes and onion rings on top. Repeat with the second half of the egg mixture. In the end, spread the grated nutmeg over the whole thing.

Nutrition: Calories: 263 Carbohydrates: 8 g

Protein: 20.3 g Fat: 24 g

61. Coconut Chia Pudding with Berries

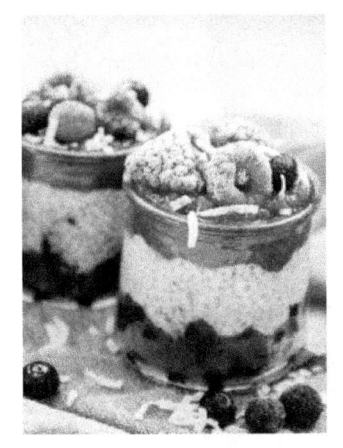

Preparation Time: 40 minutes

Cooking Time: 0 minutes

Servings: 2

Level of difficulty: Normal

Category: Green

Ingredients:

- 150 g raspberries and blueberries

- 60 g chia seeds
- 500 ml of coconut milk
- 1 teaspoon agave syrup
- ½ teaspoon ground bourbon vanilla

Directions:

1. Put the chia seeds, agave syrup, and vanilla in a bowl. Pour in the coconut milk. Mix thoroughly and let it soak for 30 minutes.
2. Meanwhile, wash the berries and let them drain well. Divide the coconut chia pudding between two glasses. Put the berries on top.

Nutrition:

Calories: 662 Carbohydrates: 18 g

Protein: 8 g Fat: 55 g

62. Eel on Scrambled Eggs and Bread

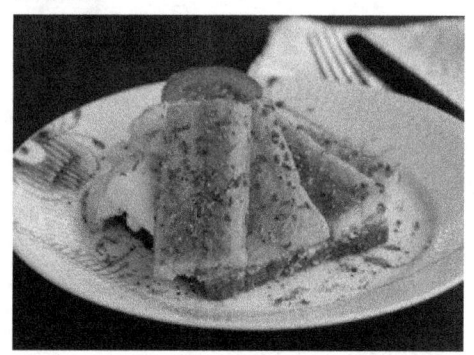

Preparation Time: 5 minutes

Cooking Time: 10 minutes

Servings: 2

Level of difficulty: Normal

Category: Lean

Ingredients:

- 4 eggs
- 1 shallot
- 4 slices of low carb bread
- 2 sticks of dill
- 200 g smoked eel
- 1 tbsp. oil
- salt
- White pepper

Directions:

1. Mix the eggs in a bowl and flavor it with salt and pepper. Peel the shallot and cut it into fine cubes. Chop the dill.
2. Remove the skin from the eel and cut it into pieces. Heat the oil in a pan and steam the shallot in it, then add the eggs and let them set. Use the spatula to turn the eggs several times.
3. Reduce the heat and add the dill, then stir everything. Spread the scrambled eggs over four slices of bread. Put the eel pieces on top. Add some fresh dill and serve everything.

Nutrition:

Calories: 830 Carbohydrates: 8 g

Protein: 45 g

Fat: 64 g

63. Chia Seed Gel with Pomegranate and Nuts

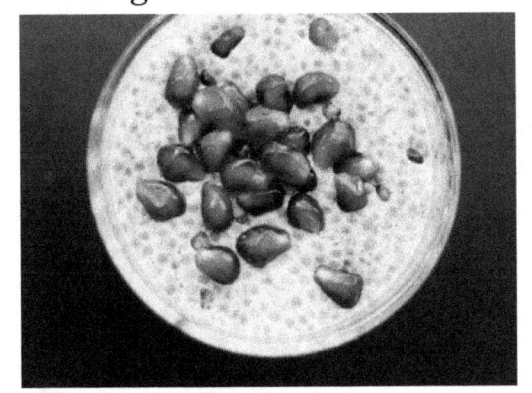

Preparation Time: 15 minutes

Cooking Time: 0 minutes

Servings: 3

Level of difficulty: Normal

Category: Healthy Fat

Ingredients:

- 20 g hazelnuts
- 20 g walnuts
- 120 ml of almond milk
- 4 tbsp. chia seeds
- 4 tbsp. pomegranate seeds
- 1 teaspoon agave syrup
- Some lime juices

Directions:

1. Finely chop the nuts. Mix the almond milk plus chia seeds. Let everything soak for 10 to 20 minutes. Occasionally stir the mixture with the chia seeds.
2. Stir in the agave syrup. Pour 2 tablespoons of each mixture into a dessert glass—Layer the chopped nuts on top.
3. Cover the nuts with 1 tablespoon each of the chia mass. Sprinkle the pomegranate seeds on top, then serve everything.

Nutrition:

Calories: 248

Carbohydrates: 7 g

Protein: 1 g

Fat: 19 g

64. Lavender Blueberry Chia Seed Pudding

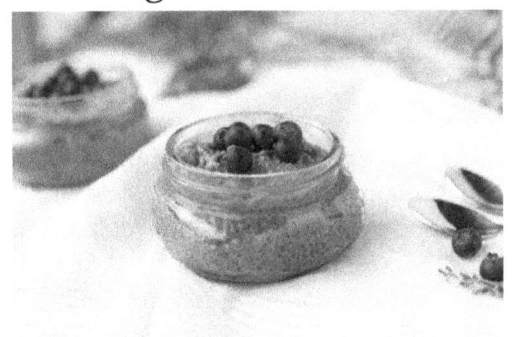

Preparation Time: 1 hour 10 minutes

Cooking Time: 0 minutes

Servings: 4

Level of difficulty: Normal

Category: Green

Ingredients:

- 100 g blueberries

- 70 g organic quark
- 50 g soy yogurt
- 30 g hazelnuts
- 200 ml of almond milk
- 2 tbsp. chia seeds
- 2 teaspoons agave syrup
- 2 teaspoons of lavender

Directions:

1. Bring the almond milk to a boil along with the lavender. Let the mixture simmer for 10 minutes at a reduced temperature.
2. Let them cool down afterward. If the milk is cold, add the blueberries and puree everything. Mix the whole thing with the chia seeds and agave syrup.
3. Let everything soak in the refrigerator for an hour. Mix the yogurt and curd cheese. Add both to the crowd. Divide the pudding into glasses. Finely chop the hazelnuts and sprinkle them on top.

Nutrition:

Calories: 252

Carbohydrates: 12 g

Protein: 1 g

Fat: 11 g

65. Yogurt with Granola and Persimmon

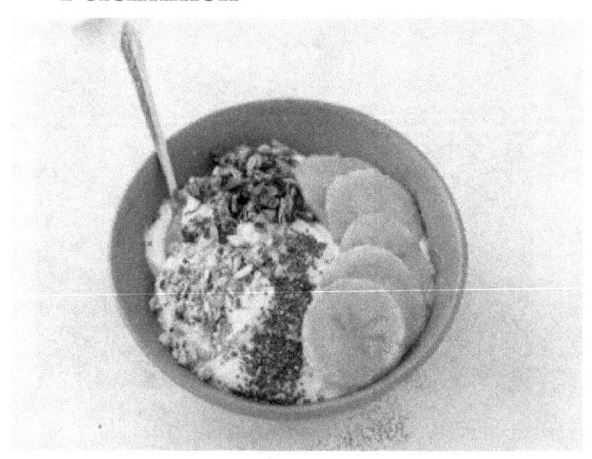

Preparation Time: 5 minutes

Cooking Time: 5 minutes

Servings: 1

Level of difficulty: Easy

Category: Leanest

Ingredients:

- 150g Greek-style yogurt
- 20g oatmeal
- 60g fresh persimmons
- 30 ml of tap water

Directions:

1. Put the oatmeal in the pan without any fat. Toast them, continually stirring, until golden brown. Then put them on a plate and let them cool down briefly.
2. Peel the persimmon and put it in a bowl with the water. Mix the whole thing into a fine puree. Put the

yogurt, the toasted oatmeal, and then puree in layers in a glass and serve.

Nutrition:

Calories: 286

Carbohydrates: 29 g

Protein: 1 g

Fat: 11 g

66. Fried Egg with Bacon

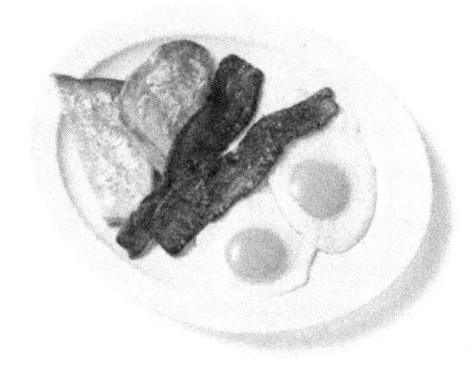

Preparation Time: 5 minutes

Cooking Time: 10 minutes

Servings: 1

Level of difficulty: Easy

Category: Lean

Ingredients:

- 2 eggs
- 30 grams of bacon
- 2 tbsp. olive oil
- salt
- pepper

Directions:

1. Heat-up oil in the pan and fry the bacon. Reduce the heat and beat the eggs in the pan. Cook the eggs and season with salt and pepper. Serve the fried eggs hot with the bacon.

Nutrition:

Calories: 405

Carbohydrates: 1 g

Protein: 19 g

Fat: 38 g

67. Whole Grain Bread and Avocado

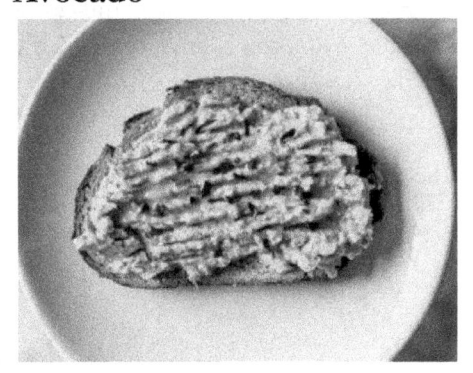

Preparation Time: 5 minutes

Cooking Time: 0 minutes

Servings: 1

Level of difficulty: Easy

Category: Healthy Fat

Ingredients:

- 2 slices of whole meal bread

- 60 g of cottage cheese
- 1 stick of thyme
- ½ avocado
- ½ lime
- Chili flakes
- salt
- pepper

Directions:

1. Cut the avocado in half. Remove the pulp and cut it into slices. Pour the lime juice over it. Wash the thyme and shake it dry.
2. Remove the leaves from the stem. Brush the whole wheat bread with cottage cheese. Place the avocado slices on top. Top with the chili flakes and thyme. Add salt and pepper and serve.

Nutrition:

Calories: 490 Carbohydrates: 31 g

Protein: 19 g Fat: 21 g

68. Porridge with Walnuts

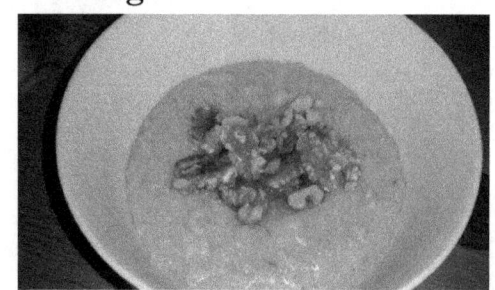

Preparation Time: 5 minutes

Cooking Time: 10 minutes

Servings: 1

Level of difficulty: Easy

Category: Healthy Fat

Ingredients:

- 50 g raspberries
- 50 g blueberries
- 25 g of ground walnuts
- 20 g of crushed flaxseed
- 10 g of oatmeal
- 200 ml nut drink
- Agave syrup
- ½ teaspoon cinnamon
- salt

Directions:

1. Warm the nut drink in a small saucepan. Add the walnuts, flaxseed, and oatmeal, stirring constantly. Stir in the cinnamon and salt.
2. Simmer for 8 minutes. Keep stirring everything. Sweet the whole thing. Put the porridge in a bowl. Wash the berries and let them drain. Add them to the porridge and serve everything.

Nutrition:

Calories: 378

Carbohydrates: 11 g

Protein: 18 g

Fat: 27 g

69. Zucchini Noodles with Creamy Avocado Pesto

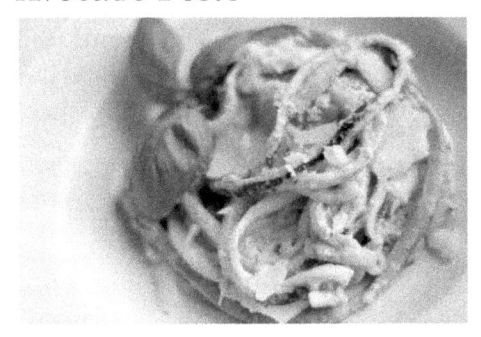

Preparation Time: 10 minutes

Cooking Time: 20 minutes

Servings: 4

Level of difficulty: Normal

Category: Green

Ingredients:

- 6 cups of spiralized zucchini
- 1 tbsp. olive oil
- 6 oz. of avocado
- 1 basil leaves
- 3 garlic cloves
- 1/3 oz. pine nuts
- 2 tbsp. lemon juice
- ½ tsp salt - ¼ tsp black pepper

Directions:

1. Spiralize the courgettes and set them aside on paper towels so that the excess water is absorbed.
2. In a food processor, put avocados, lemon juice, basil leaves, garlic, pine nuts, and sea salt and pulse until chopped. Then put olive oil in a slow stream till emulsified and creamy.
3. Drizzle olive oil in a skillet over medium-high heat and put zucchini noodles, cooking for about 2 minutes till tender.
4. Put zucchini noodles into a big bowl and toss with avocado pesto. Season with cracked pepper and a little Parmesan and serve.

Nutrition: Calories 115 Protein 30g

Fat 0g Carbs 3g

70. Avocado Chicken Salad

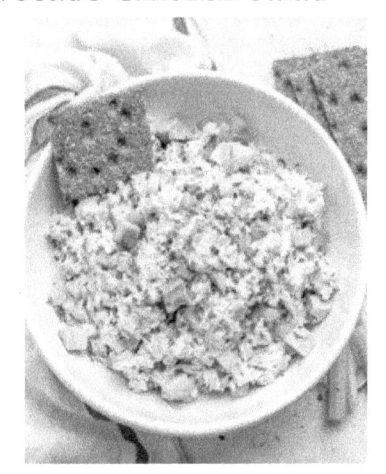

Preparation Time: 5 minutes

Cooking Time: 10 minutes

Servings: 2

Level of difficulty: Easy

Category: Leaner

Ingredients:

- 10 oz. diced cooked chicken

- ½ cup 2% Plain Greek yogurt
- 3 oz. chopped avocado
- 12 tsp garlic powder
- ¼ tsp salt
- 1/8 tsp pepper
- 1 tbsp. + 1 tsp lime juice
- ¼ cup fresh cilantro, chopped

Directions:

1. Combine all ingredients in a medium-sized bowl. Refrigerate until ready to serve. Cut the chicken salad in half and serve with your favorite greens.

Nutrition:

Calories 265

Protein 35g

Fat 13g

Carbs 5g

CHAPTER 6:

Main Dishes

71. Baked Ricotta with Pears

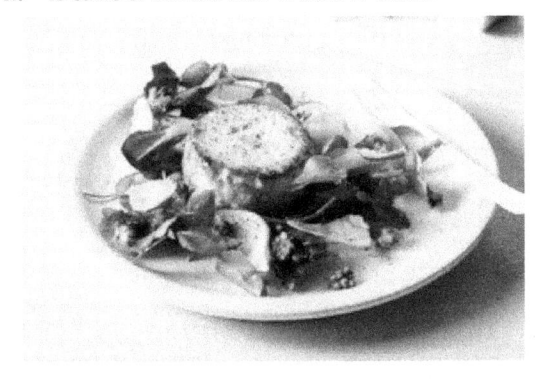

Preparation time: 5 minutes

Cooking time: 25 minutes

Servings: 4

Level of difficulty: Normal

Category: Green

Ingredients:

- Nonstick cooking spray
- 1 (16-ounce) container whole-milk ricotta cheese
- 2 large eggs
- 1/4 cup white whole-wheat flour
- 1 tablespoon sugar
- 1 teaspoon vanilla extract
- 1/4 teaspoon ground nutmeg
- 1 pear, cored and diced
- 2 tablespoons water
- 1 tablespoon honey

Directions:

1. Preheat the oven to 400°F. Oiled four 6-ounce ramekins with nonstick cooking spray. Beat the ricotta, eggs, flour, sugar, vanilla, and nutmeg in a large bowl. Spoon into the ramekins.
2. Bake for 22 to 25 minutes, or until the ricotta is just about set. Remove from the oven and cool slightly on racks.
3. While the ricotta is baking, in a small saucepan over medium heat, simmer the pear in the water for 10 minutes, until slightly softened.
4. Remove, then stir in the honey. Serve the ricotta ramekins topped with the warmed pear.

Nutrition:

Calories: 312

Fat: 17g

Carbohydrates: 23g

Protein: 17g

72. Herbed Wild Rice

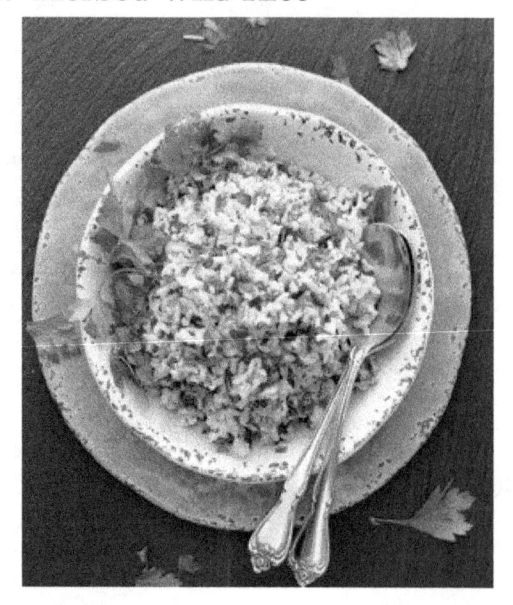

Preparation time: 10 minutes

Cooking time: 4-6 hours

Servings: 8

Level of difficulty: Normal

Category: Green

Ingredients:

- 3 cups wild rice, rinsed and drained
- 6 cups Vegetable Broth
- 1 onion, chopped
- 1/2 teaspoon salt
- 1/2 teaspoon dried thyme leaves
- 1/2 teaspoon dried basil leaves
- 1 bay leaf
- 1/3 cup chopped fresh flat-leaf parsley

Directions:

1. In a 6-quart slow cooker, mix the wild rice, vegetable broth, onion, salt, thyme, basil, and bay leaf. Cover and cook on low for 4 to 6 hours, or until the wild rice is tender but still firm.
2. You can cook this dish longer until the wild rice pops, taking about 7 to 8 hours. Remove and discard the bay leaf. Stir in the parsley and serve.

Nutrition:

Calories: 258 Carbohydrates: 54 g

Fat: 2 g Protein: 6 g

73. Buffalo Chicken Sliders

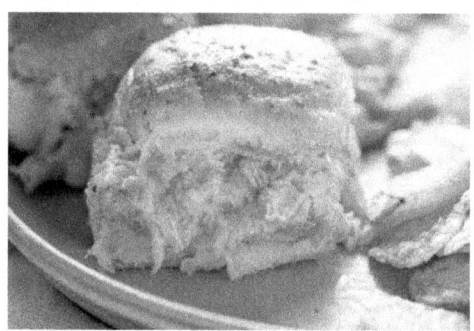

Preparation time: 10 minutes

Cooking time: 15 minutes

Servings: 12

Level of difficulty: Normal

Category: Leaner

Ingredients:

- 2 lb. Chicken breasts, cooked, shredded
- 1 cup Wing sauce

- 1 pack Ranch dressing mix
- ¼ cup Blue cheese dressing, low fat
- Lettuce, for topping
- 12 Buns, slider

Directions:

1. Add the chicken breasts (shredded, cooked) in a large bowl along with the ranch dressing and wing sauce. Stir well to incorporate, then place a piece of lettuce onto each slider roll.
2. Top off using the chicken mixture. Drizzle blue cheese dressing over chicken, then top off using top buns of slider rolls. Serve.

Nutrition:

Calories: 330 Carbs: 32g

Fat: 6g Protein: 35g

74. High Protein Chicken Meatballs

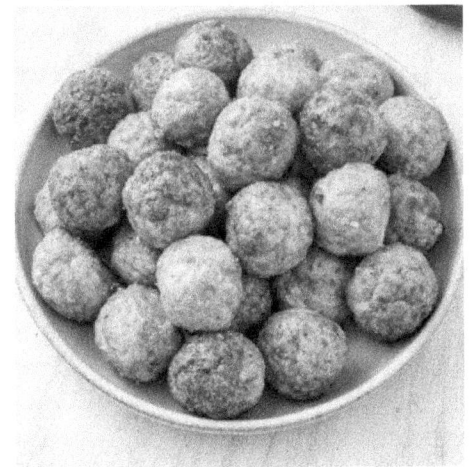

Preparation time: 5 minutes

Cooking time: 25 minutes

Servings: 2

Level of difficulty: Normal

Category: Lean

Ingredients:

- 1 lb. Chicken, lean, ground
- ¾ cup Oats rolled
- 2 Onions, grated
- 2 tsp Allspice, ground
- Salt and black pepper

Directions:

1. Heat a skillet (large) over medium heat, then grease using cooking spray. Add in the onions (grated), chicken (lean, ground), oats (rolled), allspice (earth), and a dash of salt and black pepper in a large-sized bowl, stir well to incorporate.
2. Shape mixture into meatballs (small). Place into the skillet (greased). Cook for roughly within 5 minutes until golden brown on all sides. Remove meatballs from heat, then serve immediately.

Nutrition:

Calories: 519

Protein: 57g

Carbohydrates: 32 g

Fat :15 g

75. Barley Risotto

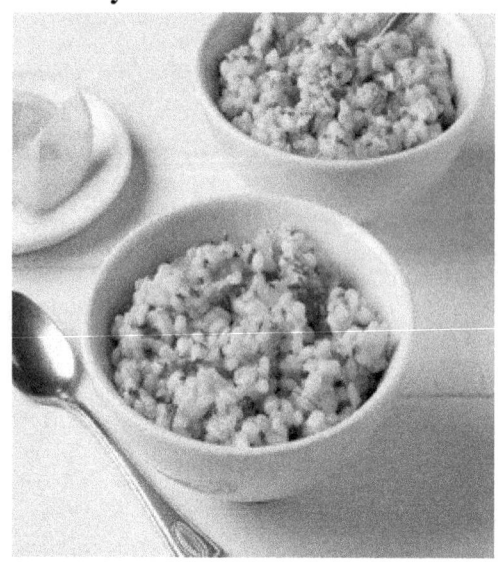

Preparation time: 15 minutes

Cooking time: 7-8 hours

Servings: 8

Level of difficulty: Normal

Category: Green

Ingredients:

- 2 1/4 cups hulled barley, rinsed
- 1 onion, finely chopped
- 4 garlic cloves, minced
- 1 (8-ounce) package button mushrooms, chopped
- 6 cups low-sodium vegetable broth
- 1/2 teaspoon dried marjoram leaves
- 1/8 teaspoon freshly ground black pepper
- 2/3 cup grated Parmesan cheese

Directions:

1. In a 6-quart slow cooker, mix the barley, onion, garlic, mushrooms, broth, marjoram, and pepper.
2. Cover and cook on low within 7 to 8 hours, or until the barley has absorbed most of the liquid and is tender, and the vegetables are tender. Stir in the Parmesan cheese and serve.

Nutrition: Calories: 288 Carbohydrates: 45 g

Fat: 6 g Protein: 13 g

76. Risotto with Green Beans, Sweet Potatoes, And Peas

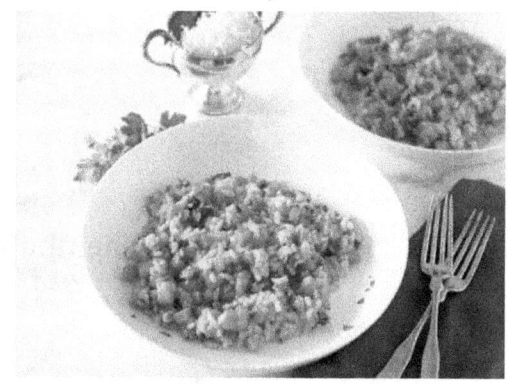

Preparation time: 20 minutes

Cooking time: 4-5 hours

Servings: 8

Level of difficulty: Normal

Category: Green

Ingredients:

- 1 large sweet potato, peeled and chopped

- 1 onion, chopped
- 5 garlic cloves, minced
- 2 cups short-grain brown rice
- 1 teaspoon dried thyme leaves
- 7 cups low-sodium vegetable broth
- 2 cups green beans, cut in half crosswise
- 2 cups frozen baby peas
- 3 tablespoons unsalted butter
- 1/2 cup grated Parmesan cheese

Directions:

1. In a 6-quart slow cooker, mix the sweet potato, onion, garlic, rice, thyme, and broth. 2Cover and cook on low for 3 to 4 hours, or until the rice is tender.
2. Stir in the green beans plus frozen peas. Cover and cook on low for 30 to 40 minutes or until the vegetables are tender. Stir in the butter and cheese. Cover and cook on low for 20 minutes, then stir and serve.

Nutrition:

Calories: 385

Carbohydrates: 52 g

Fat: 10 g

Protein: 10 g

77. Maple Lemon Tempeh Cubes

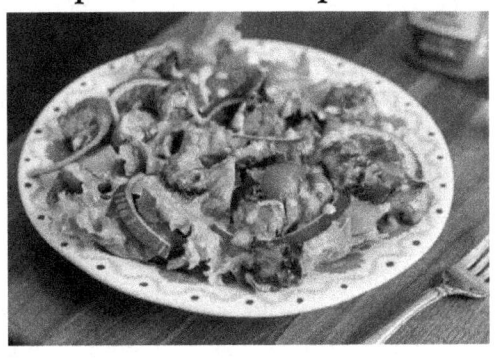

Preparation time: 10 minutes

Cooking time: 30-40 minutes

Servings: 4

Level of difficulty: Normal

Category: Green

Ingredients:

- 1 packet tempeh
- 2-3 tsp coconut oil
- 3 tbsp lemon juice
- 2 tsp maple syrup
- 1-2 tsp Bragg's liquid aminos or low-sodium tamari (optional)
- 2 tsp water
- ¼ tsp dried basil
- ¼ tsp powdered garlic
- black pepper (freshly grounded); to taste

Directions:

1. Heat your oven to 400 ° C. Cut your tempeh block into squares in bite

form. Heat coconut oil over medium to high heat in a nonstick skillet.

2. When melted and heated, add the tempeh and cook on one side for 2-4 minutes, or until the tempeh turns down into a golden-brown color.

3. Flip the tempeh bits, and cook for 2-4 minutes. Mix the lemon juice, tamari, maple syrup, basil, water, garlic, and black pepper while tempeh is browning.

4. Drop the mixture over tempeh, then swirl to cover the tempeh. Sauté for 2-3 minutes, then turn the tempeh and sauté 1-2 minutes more. The tempeh, on both sides, should be soft and orange. Serve.

Nutrition: Calories: 22 Fats: 17 g

Carbs: 5 g Protein: 21 g

78. Bok Choy With Tofu Stir Fry

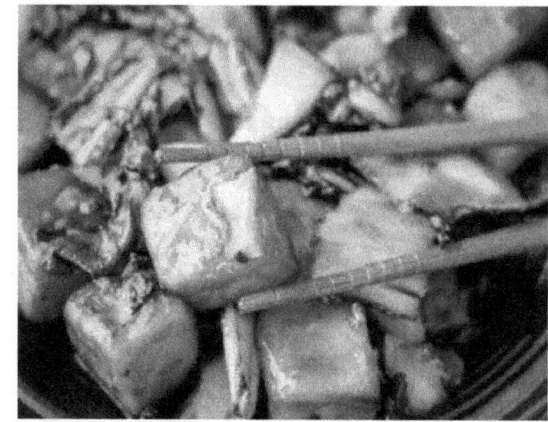

Preparation time: 15 minutes

Cooking time: 15 minutes

Servings: 4

Level of difficulty: Normal

Category: Green

Ingredients:

- 1 lb. super-firm tofu drained and pressed
- 1 tbsp coconut oil
- 1 clove of garlic, minced
- 3 heads baby bok choy, chopped
- low-sodium vegetable broth
- 2 tsp maple syrup
- braggs liquid aminos
- 1-2 tsp chili sauce
- 1 scallion or green onion, chopped
- 1 tsp grated ginger
- quinoa/rice, for serving

Directions:

1. With paper towels, Pat pressed the tofu dry and cut into tiny pieces of bite-size around 1/2 inch wide.

2. Heat coconut oil in a wide skillet onto a warm. Remove tofu and stir-fry until painted softly. Stir-fry for 1-2 minutes before the choy of the Bok starts to wilt.

3. When this occurs, you'll want to apply the vegetable broth and all the remaining ingredients to the skillet.

4. Hold the mixture stir-frying until all components are well coated and the bulk of the liquid evaporates, around

5-6 minutes. Serve over brown rice or quinoa.

Nutrition: Calories: 263.7 Fat 4.2 g

Protein: 0 g Carbohydrate: 35.7 g

79. Three-Bean Medley

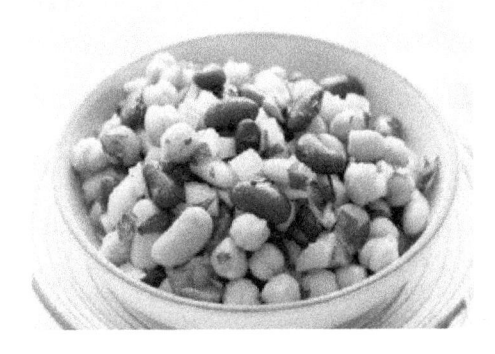

Preparation time: 15 minutes

Cooking time: 6-8 hours

Servings: 8

Level of difficulty: Easy

Category: Green

Ingredients:

- 1 1/4 cups dried kidney beans, rinsed and drained
- 1 1/4 cups dried black beans, rinsed and drained
- 1 1/4 cups dried black-eyed peas, rinsed and drained
- 1 onion, chopped
- 1 leek, chopped
- 2 garlic cloves, minced
- 2 carrots, peeled and chopped
- 6 cups low-sodium vegetable broth
- 1 1/2 cups water
- 1/2 teaspoon dried thyme leaves

Directions:

1. In a 6-quart slow cooker, mix all of the ingredients. Cover and cook on low for 6 to 8 hours, or until the beans are tender and the liquid is absorbed. Serve.

Nutrition: Calories: 284 Carbohydrates: 56 g

Fat: 0 g Protein: 1 9g

80. Herbed Garlic Black Beans

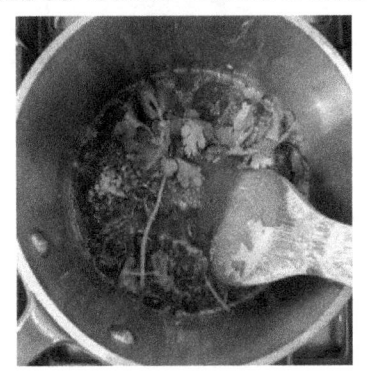

Preparation time: 10 minutes

Cooking time: 7-9 hours

Servings: 8

Level of difficulty: Easy

Category: Green

Ingredients:

- 3 cups dried black beans, rinsed and drained

- 2 onions, chopped
- 8 garlic cloves, minced
- 6 cups low-sodium vegetable broth
- 1/2 teaspoon salt
- 1 teaspoon dried basil leaves
- 1/2 teaspoon dried thyme leaves
- 1/2 teaspoon dried oregano leaves

Directions:

1. In a 6-quart slow cooker, mix all the ingredients. Cover and cook on low within 7 to 9 hours, or until the beans have absorbed the liquid and are tender. Remove and discard the bay leaf. Serve.

Nutrition:

Calories: 250 Carbohydrates: 47 g

Fat: 0 g Protein: 15 g

81. Quinoa with Vegetables

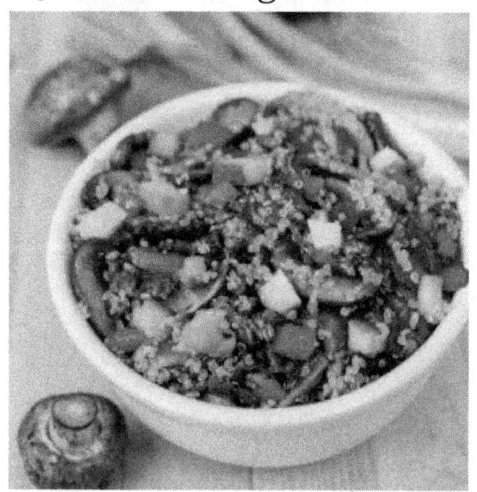

Preparation time: 10 minutes

Cooking time: 5-6 hours

Servings: 8

Level of difficulty: Easy

Category: Green

Ingredients:

- 2 cups quinoa, rinsed and drained
- 2 onions, chopped
- 2 carrots, peeled and sliced
- 1 cup sliced cremini mushrooms
- 3 garlic cloves, minced
- 4 cups low-sodium vegetable broth
- 1/2 teaspoon salt
- 1 teaspoon dried marjoram leaves
- 1/8 teaspoon freshly ground black pepper

Directions:

1. In a 6-quart slow cooker, mix all of the ingredients. Cover and cook on low for 5 to 6 hours, or until the quinoa and vegetables are tender. Stir the mixture and serve.

Nutrition:

Calories: 204

Carbohydrates: 35 g

Fat: 3 g

Protein: 7 g

82. Pan-Fried Salmon

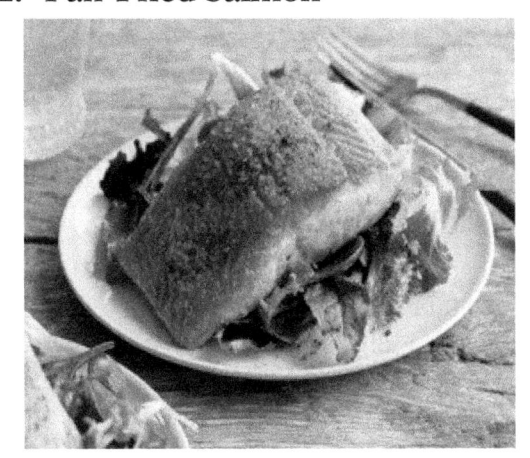

Preparation time: 5 minutes

Cooking time: 20 minutes

Servings: 4

Level of difficulty: Normal

Category: Lean

Ingredients:

- 4 salmon fillets
- 1 teaspoon dried oregano
- Salt and pepper
- 3 tbsp olive oil
- 1 tsp dried basil

Directions:

1. Marinate the fish with pepper, oregano, salt, and basil. Warm the oil in a pan and put the salmon in the cooking oil.
2. Fry on per side for around 2 minutes until it turns golden brown and odorous. Serve the salmon fresh and warm.

Nutrition: Calories: 327 Fat: 25g

Protein: 36g Carbohydrates: 0.3g

83. Mediterranean Chickpea Salad

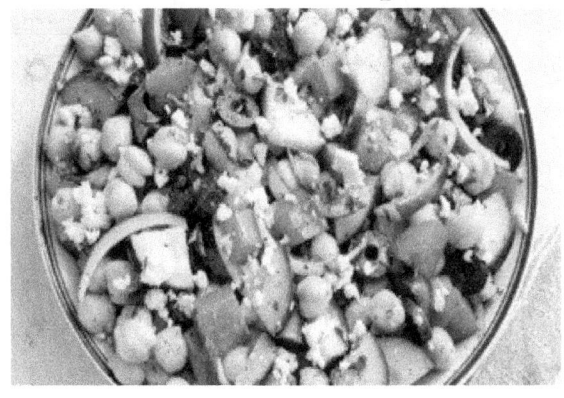

Preparation time: 5 minutes

Cooking time: 20 minutes

Servings: 6

Level of difficulty: Easy

Category: Green

Ingredients:

- 1 red onion, sliced
- 1 can chickpeas, drained
- 1 teaspoon dried oregano
- chopped parsley (2 tablespoons)
- 1 teaspoon dried basil
- 1 fennel bulb, sliced
- 2 tablespoons lemon juice
- 2 tbsp olive oil
- Salt

- 4 garlic cloves, minced
- pepper

Directions:

1. Add the chickpeas, oil, red onion, fennel, herbs, lemon juice, and garlic in a bowl. Mix pepper and salt. Serve.

Nutrition: Calories: 200 Fat: 9g

Protein: 4g Carbohydrates: 28g

84. Zucchini Salmon Salad

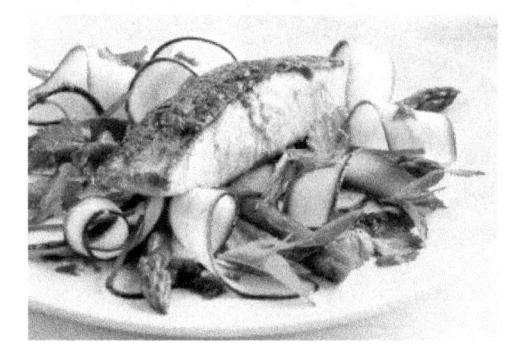

Preparation time: 5 minutes

Cooking time: 10 minutes

Servings: 3

Level of difficulty: Normal

Category: Lean

Ingredients:

- 2 salmon fillets
- pepper and salt
- 2 tbsp soy sauce (2 tablespoons)
- 2 tablespoons olive oil
- 2 zucchinis, sliced
- 2 tablespoons sesame seeds

Directions:

1. Mix the salmon with soy sauce. Heat a grill vessel to medium flame. Cook salmon on the grill and heat per side for around 2-3 minutes
2. Marinate the zucchini with pepper and salt and put it on the grill as well as salmon. Cook on per side until golden brown. Place the salmon, zucchini, and the rest of the components in a bowl. Serve.

Nutrition: Calories: 224 Fat: 19g

Protein: 18g Carbohydrates: 0g

85. Greek Roasted Fish

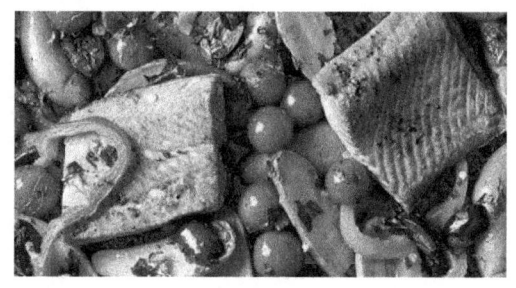

Preparation time: 5 minutes

Cooking time: 30 minutes

Servings: 4

Category: Lean

Level of difficulty: Easy

Ingredients:

- 4 salmon fillets
- 2 tbsp olive oil

- 1 teaspoon dried basil
- 1 red onion, sliced
- 1 tablespoon chopped oregano
- 1 carrot, sliced
- 1 zucchini, sliced
- 1 lemon, sliced
- Salt and pepper

Directions:

1. Preheat the oven to 350F. Mix all the components to the baking pan. Add pepper and salt and then cook for around 20 minutes. Serve the vegetables and fish warm.

Nutrition: Calories: 328 Fat: 13g

Protein: 38g Carbohydrates: 8g

86. Oregano Pork Mix

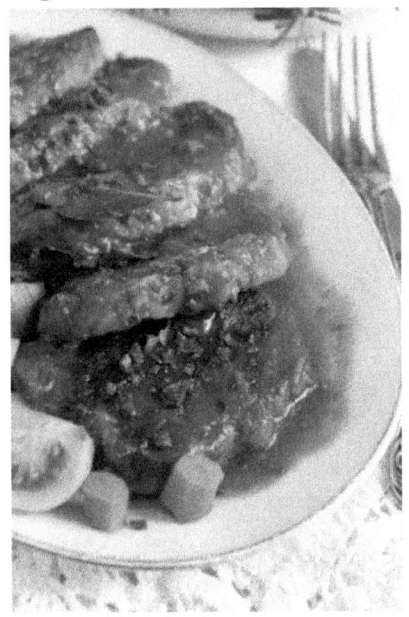

Preparation time: 5 minutes

Cooking time: 7 hours & 6 minutes

Servings: 5

Level of difficulty: Normal

Category: Lean

Ingredients:

- 1 yellow onion, chopped
- 2 pounds' pork roast
- 1 cup beef stock
- olive oil (2 tablespoons)
- 2 tablespoons fresh oregano chopped
- 1 tablespoon garlic, minced
- 2 tablespoons ground cumin
- ½ cup fresh thyme, chopped
- 7 ounces' tomato paste

Directions:

1. Heat a saucepan with the oil over average temperature. Add the roast and brown it for around 3 minutes per side. Then shift to your slow cooker.
2. Add the rest of the components and stir—Cook at a low temperature for around 7 hours. Slice the roast, distribute it between plates.

Nutrition:

Calories 623 Carbs 19.3 g

Fat 30.1 g Protein 69.2 g

87. Simple Beef Roast

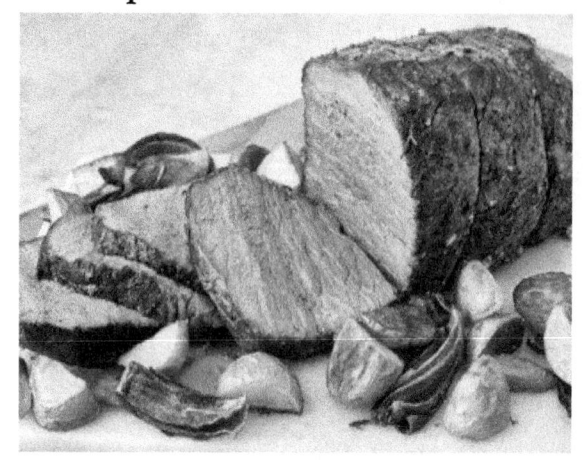

Preparation time: 10 minutes

Cooking time: 8 hours

Servings: 8

Level of difficulty: Normal

Category: Lean

Ingredients:

- 5 pounds' beef roast
- 1 cup beef stock
- 3 tbsp olive oil
- 1 tbsp sweet paprika
- 2 tablespoons Italian seasoning

Directions:

1. Mix all the components in your slow cooker. Lid it, and cook on low temperature for 8 hours. Slice the roast, divide it between plates. Serve them and enjoy

Nutrition: Calories 587 Fat 24.1g

Carbs 0.9g Protein 86.5g

88. Pork and Peppers Chili

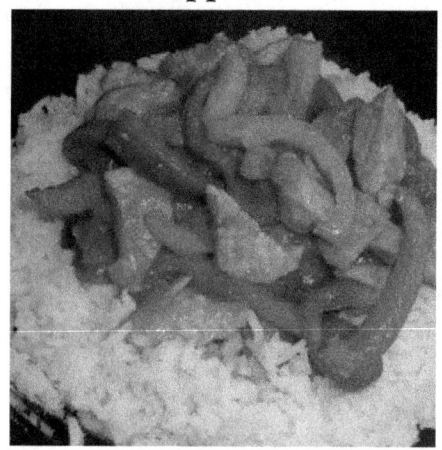

Preparation time: 5 minutes

Cooking time: 8 hours & 5 minutes

Servings: 4

Level of difficulty: Normal

Category: Lean

Ingredients:

- 2 pounds' pork
- 2 red bell peppers, chopped
- 4 garlic cloves, minced
- 1 red onion, chopped
- 25 ounces' fresh tomatoes crushed
- ¼ cup green chilies, chopped
- 1 celery stalk, chopped
- A pinch of black pepper and salt
- fresh oregano chopped (olive oil 2 tablespoons)
- 2 tablespoons chili powder

Directions:

1. Heat a saucepan with the oil above medium temperature. Add the garlic, onion, and meat, mix them well and put aside.
2. Cook for 5 minutes, and then transfer to your slow cooker. Add the rest of the Components. Lid it and cook on low for 8 hours. Distribute everything into bowls.

Nutrition: Calories 448 Carbs 20.2 g

Fat 13 gProtein 63 g

89. Chicken Breast Soup

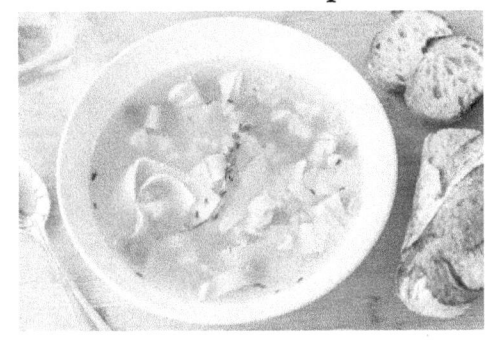

Preparation time: 5 minutes

Cooking time: 4 hours

Servings: 4

Level of difficulty: Normal

Category: Leaner

Ingredients:

- 2 celery stalks, chopped
- 2 tbsp olive oil
- 3 chicken breasts, boneless and cubed
- 1 red onion, chopped
- 4 cups chicken stock
- 3 garlic cloves, minced
- 2 carrots, chopped
- 1 tbsp parsley, chopped

Directions:

1. Mix all the components except the parsley in your slow cooker. Lid it and cook on high temperature for 4 hours. Add the parsley, stir well. Ladle the soup into bowls

Nutrition: Calories 445 Carbs 7.4g

Fat 21.1g Protein 54.3g

90. Tomato Fish Bake

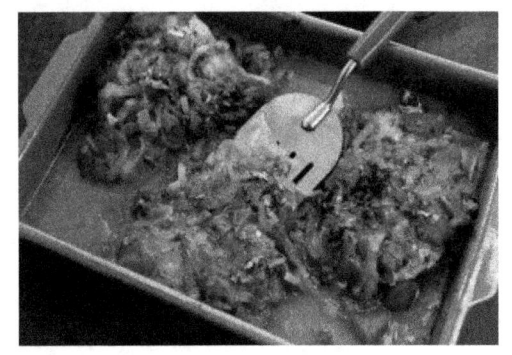

Preparation time: 5 minutes

Cooking time: 30 minutes

Servings: 4

Level of difficulty: Easy

Category: Leanest

Ingredients:

- 4 cod fillets

- 4 garlic cloves
- 1 tsp fennel seeds
- 1 celery stalk, sliced
- 4 tomatoes, sliced
- 1 cup vegetable stock
- 1 shallot, sliced
- Salt and pepper

Directions:
1. Preheat the oven to 350F. Cover the tomatoes and cod fillets in a baking pan. Add all the ingredients and add pepper and salt. Cook in the oven for around 20 minutes. Serve the dish chilled or warm.

Nutrition:

Calories: 299 Fat: 3g

Carbohydrates: 2g Protein: 64g

91. Warm Chorizo Chickpea Salad

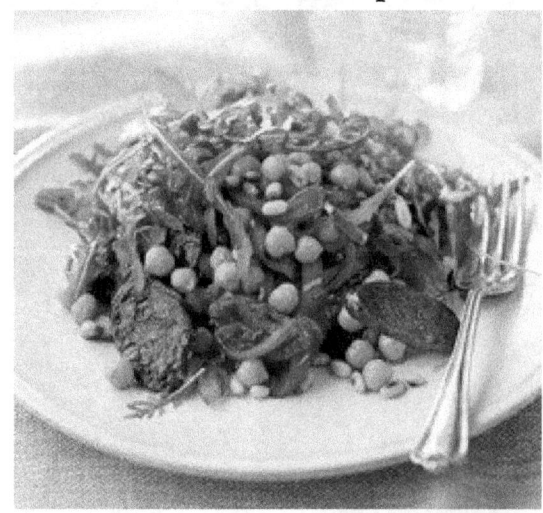

Preparation time: 5 minutes

Cooking time: 20 minutes

Servings: 6

Level of difficulty: Easy

Category: Green

Ingredients:
- 4 chorizo links, sliced
- pepper and salt
- 1 tablespoon olive oil
- 1 can chickpeas, drained
- 2 cups cherry tomatoes
- 1 red onion, sliced
- 4 roasted red bell peppers, chopped
- 2 tablespoons balsamic vinegar

Directions:
1. Cook the oil in a saucepan and add the chorizo. Cook briefly just until fragrant, and then add the bell peppers, chickpeas, and onion.
2. Cook for 2 extra minutes. Put the mixture in a salad bowl, and then add the vinegar, salt, tomatoes, and pepper. Mix them properly and serve.

Nutrition:

Calories: 359

Fat: 18g

Protein: 15g

Carbohydrates: 21g

92. Chicken Broccoli Salad with Avocado Dressing

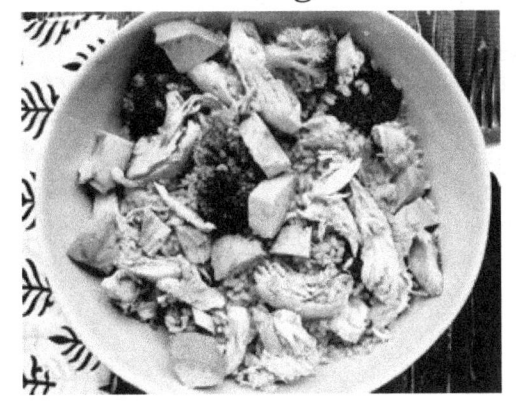

Preparation time: 5 minutes

Cooking time: 0 minutes

Servings: 1

Level of difficulty: Easy

Category: Leaner

Ingredients:

- 1-pound broccoli, cut into florets
- ¼ teaspoon cumin powder
- 2 chicken breasts
- 2 garlic cloves
- 1 avocado, peeled and pitted
- ¼ teaspoon chili powder
- ½ lemon, juiced
- pepper and salt

Directions:

1. Heat the chicken in a big pan of salty water. Remove water and chop the chicken into a small piece. Then place them in a bowl.
2. Put the broccoli and mix well. Add the lemon juice, salt, garlic, avocado, cumin powder, chili powder, and pepper in a blender and beat until smooth. Add them to the salad and mix properly. Serve.

Nutrition: Calories: 195 Fat: 11g

Protein: 14g Carbohydrates: 3g

93. Balsamic Beef and Mushrooms Mix

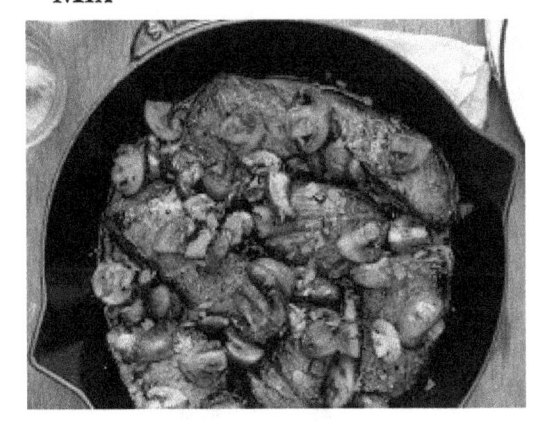

Preparation time: 5 minutes

Cooking time: 0 minutes

Servings: 1

Level of difficulty: Easy

Category: Lean

Ingredients:

- 1 cup brown mushrooms, sliced
- ¼ cup balsamic vinegar
- 1 tbsp ginger

- 1 tsp ground cinnamon
- 2 cups beef stock
- 2 pounds' beef, cut into strips
- ½ cup of lemon juice(1/2cup)
- A pinch of black pepper and salt

Directions:

1. In your slow cooker, mix all the components. Lid it and heat on low for around 8 hours. Distribute everything between plates. Serve.

Nutrition:

Calories 446

Protein 70.8g

Fat 14g

Carbs 2.9g

94. Garlicky Tomato Chicken Casserole

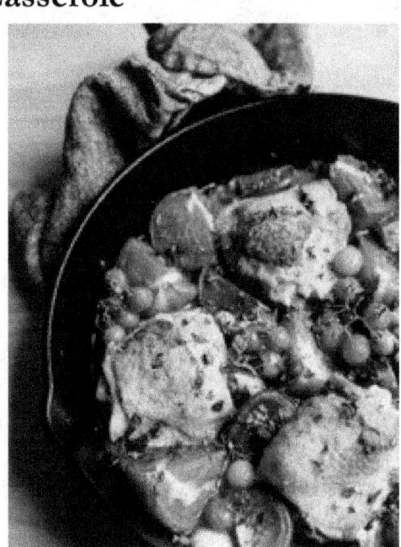

Preparation time: 5 minutes

Cooking time: 50 minutes

Servings: 4

Level of difficulty: Normal

Category: Leaner

Ingredients:

- 1 can diced tomatoes
- 4 chicken breasts
- 1 shallot, chopped
- 2 tomatoes, sliced
- 1 bay leaf
- 2 garlic cloves, chopped
- ½ cup dry white wine
- ½ cup chicken stock
- 1 thyme sprig
- pepper and salt

Directions:

1. Preheat the oven to 330F. Add the chicken and all the components to a deep bowl baking pan. Add pepper and salt.
2. Close the pot with a cover or aluminum foil, then cook them in the oven for around 40 minutes. Serve them while warm.

Nutrition:

Calories: 313 Protein: 47g

Carbohydrates: 6g Fat: 8g

95. Fennel Wild Rice Risotto

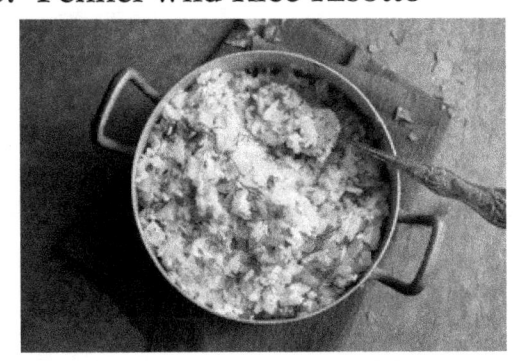

Preparation time: 5 minutes

Cooking time: 35 minutes

Servings: 6

Level of difficulty: Normal

Category: Green

Ingredients:

- 2 cups chicken stock
- 1 shallot, chopped
- 2 garlic cloves
- 2 tablespoons olive oil
- 1 fennel bulb, chopped
- 1 cup wild rice
- 1 teaspoon grated orange zest
- ¼ cup dry white wine
- pepper and salt

Directions:

1. Warm the oil in a pan. Add the shallot, fennel, and garlic. Cook them for a few minutes. Mix in the rice, heat for two extra minutes.
2. Then add the orange zest and wine, with pepper and salt to taste. Cook on low heat for around 20 minutes. Serve them while warm.

Nutrition:

Calories: 162

Protein: 8g

Fat: 2g

Carbohydrates: 20g

96. Garlic Chicken Balls

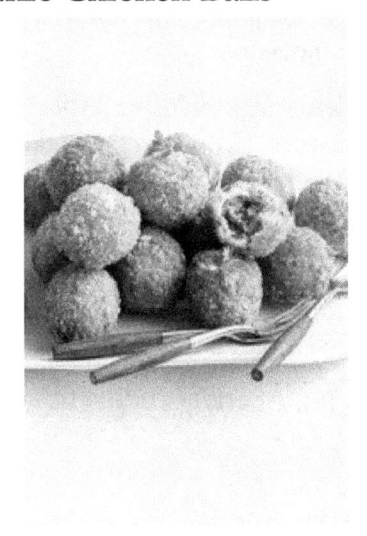

Preparation time: 5 minutes

Cooking time: 0 minutes

Servings: 1

Level of difficulty: Normal

Category: Lean

Ingredients:

- 1 teaspoon minced garlic
- 1/3 carrot, grated

- 1 egg, beaten
- 1 teaspoon dried dill
- 2 cups ground chicken
- ¼ cup coconut flakes
- ½ teaspoon salt
- 1 tbsp olive oil

Directions:

1. Mix up together minced garlic, egg, dried dill, ground chicken, carrot, and salt in a bowl. Mash the chicken with the help of the fingertips until homogenous.
2. Then make average balls from the mixture. Cover every chicken ball in coconut flakes—heat olive oil in the skillet. Put chicken balls into the oil; cook them for 3 minutes from each side or brownish color.

Nutrition: Calories 200 Carbs 1.7g

Fat 11.5g Protein 21.9g

97. Sliced Steak with Canadian Crust

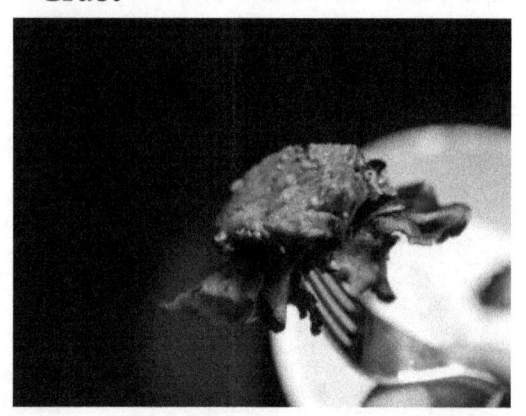

Preparation Time: 10 minutes

Cooking Time: 20 minutes

Servings: 5

Level of difficulty: Normal

Category: Lean

Ingredients:

- 2- 10-ounce steaks, about 1 and one-half thick
- 1 tablespoon dry steak seasonings

Directions

1. Preheat broiler. Rub on both sides of the steak the dry steak seasonings. Place steak under a preheated broiler.
2. Broil each side to taste within 5 minutes per side for medium-rare—slice steak in thin, 3/4" slices against the grain.
3. Arrange slices on a serving platter and top with a generous amount of butter. Serve and enjoy with a side salad.

Nutrition:

Calories: 51

Protein: 6.58 g

Fat: 2.02 g

Carbohydrates: 1.03 g

98. Fork Tender Beef Goulash with Peppercorn & Sage

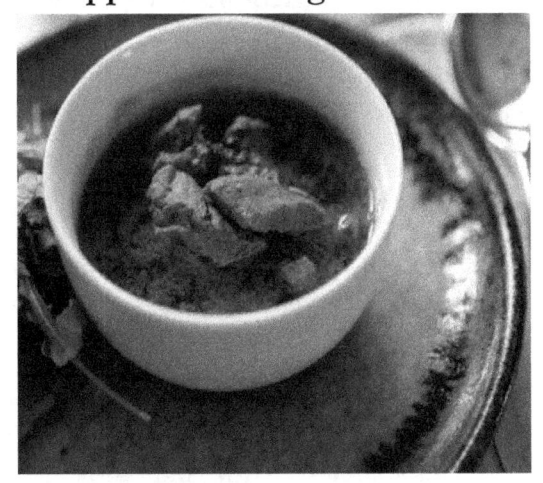

Preparation Time: 15 minutes

Cooking Time: 35 minutes

Servings: 4

Level of difficulty: Normal

Category: Lean

Ingredients:

- 2 tbsp olive oil
- 2 onions, chopped roughly
- 4 garlic cloves, crushed
- 2 celery stalks, sliced
- 800 g beef rump steaks, or use stewing steak, cut into 3cm cubes
- 1 tbsp paprika
- ½ bottle red wine
- 1 tin chopped tomato, approx. 420g
- 1 tbsp balsamic vinegar
- 1/2 peppercorn
- 2 tsp brown sugar
- 1 stalk sage, leaves only
- 1 pinch chili flakes
- 1 pottle sour cream, for serving

Directions:

1. In a heavy saucepan, sauté the onion, celery, and garlic till soft. Add the meat and brown well.
2. Set aside a small amount of the meat, sliced thinly, and return the rest to the pan along with the paprika, wine, chopped tomatoes, balsamic vinegar, and sugar.
3. Preheat the oven to 160°C. Gently simmer for 20–30 minutes, adding the whole peppercorn and sage bundle. With a sharp knife, remove the peppercorn and sage.
4. Increase the heat and simmer vigorously for another 10 minutes. Serve garnished with the reserved meat slices, sour cream, and chili flakes.

Nutrition:

Calories: 417

Protein: 44.36 g

Fat: 18.21 g

Carbohydrates: 17.78 g

99. Mexican Chicken in Orange Juice

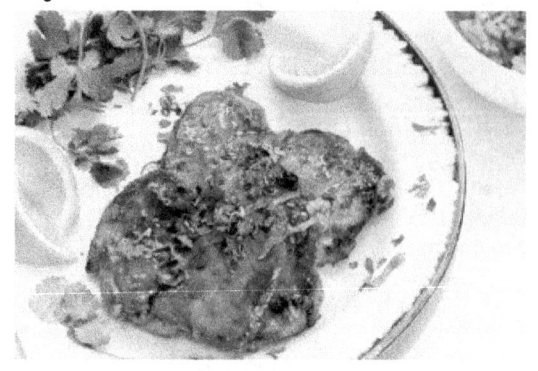

Preparation Time: 2 hours

Cooking Time: 20 minutes

Level of difficulty: Normal

Servings: 4

Category: Leaner

Ingredients

- 1 cup fresh orange juice
- 2 tbsp. fresh lime juice
- 1 dried chipotle chili pepper, stemmed and seeded
- 1 cup mild salsa
- 1/4 c. olive oil
- 1 tsp. salt
- 4 boneless, skinless chicken breast halves
- 1 orange, sliced into rings
- 1/4 cup chopped fresh cilantro leaves

Directions

1. Place all ingredients except chicken and orange slices in the blender. Blend until smooth. Store in refrigerator overnight to allow flavors to blend.
2. Add chicken to orange juice mixture and marinate for 2 hours. Prepare grill for medium heat. Remove chicken from marinade; reserve marinade.
3. Place chicken on grill rack coated with nonstick cooking spray and grill 10 minutes. Turn and cook until juices run clear. Move the chicken to your cutting board, then cut into thin bite-size slices.
4. Pour reserved marinade into a small saucepan. Boil it on high heat, then adjust the heat to medium and boil for 5 minutes. Add orange slices to the saucepan and mix well. Heat through.
5. Divide cilantro evenly among 4 dinner plates. Top each of the plates evenly with orange slices and sauced chicken. Garnish with lime slices and serve.
6. Nutrition:

Calories: 489

Protein: 55.23 g

Fat: 19.98 g

Carbohydrates: 20.47 g

100. Chicken Sancho

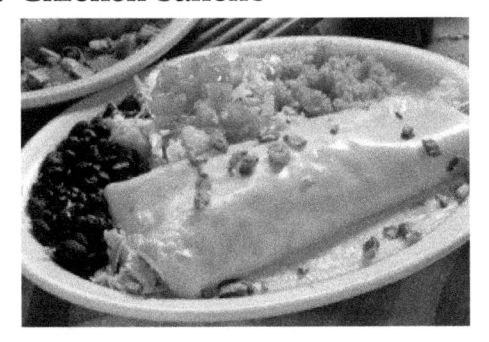

Preparation Time: 5 minutes

Cooking Time: 1 hour

Servings: 6

Level of difficulty: Normal

Category: Leaner

Ingredients:

- 1 teaspoon olive oil
- 5 scallions, chopped
- 1 tomato, chopped
- 4 cloves garlic, chopped
- 1/2 onion, chopped
- 6 skinless chicken thighs on the bone
- 1 cup chopped cilantro
- 3 medium potatoes, peeled and chopped into 2-inch pieces
- 1 small green plantain, peeled & chopped into 1" pieces
- 1 tsp cumin
- 2 chicken bouillon cubes
- salt to taste

Directions:

1. Heat the oil in a large skillet, brown the chicken, skin side first over medium heat for 2-3 minutes, then take them out.
2. Preheat the oven to 350F. Chop the scallions, tomatoes, onions, and garlic in a food processor
3. Heat the skillet and add the scallion, onion, and garlic; cook for a minute or until the onion is translucent. Add the cilantro and chicken, stir.
4. Prepare the chicken broth by adding the chicken bouillon cubes to a large saucepan and adding 2 cups of water. Bring to a boil, reduce the heat and simmer for 5 min until it is fully dissolved.
5. Add the potatoes, yucca, corn, and plantain to the skillet, stir. Pour in the chicken broth, then cook until the vegetables are tender. Add a pinch or two of salt to taste.
6. Prepare the Arroz con coco (rice with coconut milk). Add 1/2 cup of the coconut milk to rice and cook according to the directions.
7. Add the chicken mixture into the rice and mix well. Garnish with cilantro.

Nutrition:

Calories: 552 Protein: 37.75 g

Fat: 38.68 g Carbohydrates: 134.47 g

CHAPTER 7:

Sides

101. Caramelized Onion Quesadilla

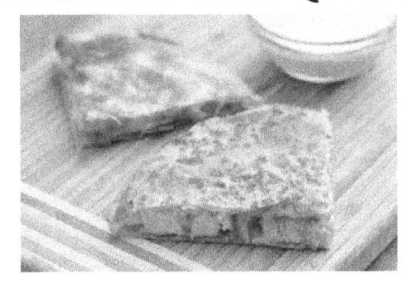

Preparation Time: 10 minutes

Cooking Time: 25 minutes

Servings: 4

Level of difficulty: Normal

Category: Green

Ingredients:

- A whole grain of tortilla
- 1 big caramelize onion, slice
- 1 cup of fresh spinach
- Black beans - Cheese (Nonfat)

Directions:

1. On medium heat, heat the onion, use dry sautéing to caramelize. Add a pinch of salt so that it can bring the moisture out of the onion.
2. Cook it until the color changes to brown and translucent, then set it aside. Heat your tortilla in a skillet. Then add your beans, spinach, and onion mixture on one side of the tortilla. Add your cheese and fold over the tortilla. Serve.

Nutrition: Calories: 350 Protein: 13.9 g

Carbohydrates: 40.9 g Fat: 26 g

102. Roasted Garlic Potatoes

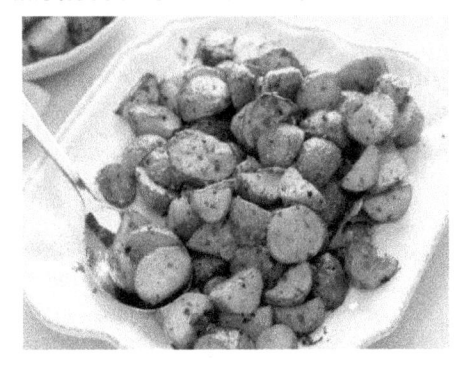

Preparation Time: 5 minutes

Cooking Time: 1 hour

Servings: 6

Level of difficulty: Normal

Category: Green

Ingredients:

- 1 teaspoon of dried or fresh chopped rosemary

- 6 cups of potatoes, unpeeled
- 1 teaspoon of onion powder
- 1 teaspoon of pepper, freshly ground

Directions:

1. Preheat the oven to 425°F. Toss the potatoes and mix with rosemary, garlic, onion powder, salt, and pepper to coat.
2. On an even layer over the already prepared baking sheet, spread the potatoes and bake for 20 minutes.
3. Stir potatoes to promote even browning of the potatoes. Continue for about 3 to 10 minutes until the potato becomes browner and more tender. Remove from the oven and serve it warm.

Nutrition: Calories: 100 Protein: 2.8 g

Carbohydrates: 23.5 g Fat: 7.9 g

103. Asian Noodle Salad

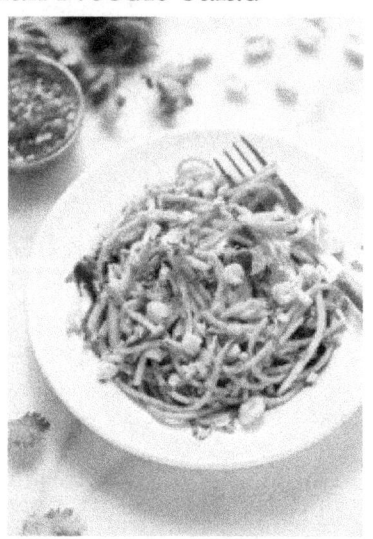

Preparation Time: 20 minutes

Cooking Time: 5 minutes

Servings: 12

Level of difficulty: Normal

Category: Green

Ingredients:

- Whole wheat of noodles, e.g., spaghetti/soba
- 24 ounces of Mann's broccoli
- 5 grated carrots
- 1/4 cup of EVOO or any preferred oil
- 1/5 cup of rice vinegar
- 4 tablespoons of honey
- 4 tablespoons of creamy butter
- 1 tablespoon mashed garlic
- 3/4 cup roasted peanuts roughly chopped

Directions:

1. Cook and drain the noodles. If you are using soba noodles, you should add a tablespoon of salt to your water, and salt won't be necessary when using Chinese noodles.
2. After draining the noodles, rinse with cold water and then spread out the noodles on a pan to dry. Steam the broccoli by viding it in boiled water and steam for about 4 minutes, rinse with cold water, and set aside.

3. In your mixing bowl, whisk together the olive or cooking oil, honey, rice vinegar, creamy butter, ginger, and garlic.

4. Pour it inside the noodle and toss. Then add the roasted peanuts at this point and toss it again. Serve chilled or at room temperature.

Nutrition:

Calories: 175

Fats: 10.6 g

Carbohydrates: 18.3 g

Protein: 3.9 g

104. Protein Pumpkin Spiced Donuts

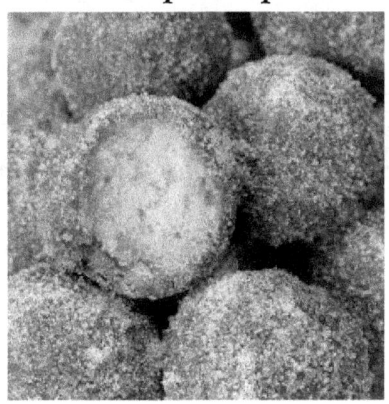

Preparation Time: 10 minutes

Cooking Time: 25 minutes

Servings: 8

Level of difficulty: Normal

Category: Green

Ingredients:

- 1 cup oat flour
- 3/4 cup xylitol
- 1 scoop, powdered vanilla protein
- 1 tbsp ground flaxseed
- 1 tbsp ground cinnamon
- 2 tsp. baking powder
- 1 tsp sea salt
- 3 beaten eggs
- 1/2 cup canned pumpkin
- 1 tbsp coconut oil, melted
- 2 tsp vanilla
- 1 tsp apple cider vinegar

Ingredients for the frosting:

- ½ cup Cream cheese, whipped
- ½ tsp Liquid stevia

Directions:

1. Place the xylitol, oat flour, ground flaxseed, powdered protein, baking powder, ground cinnamon, and a dash of sea salt in a large bowl. Preheat your oven to 350 degrees Fahrenheit.

2. Add the egg (beaten) into another bowl (large) along with the pumpkin (canned), pure vanilla and vinegar, and coconut oil (melted).

3. Whisk until mixed (evenly), then pour the mixture into the flour. Stir until thoroughly mixed. Use a cooking spray, grease a large donut pan.

4. Pour batter into the donut pan (greased). Place batter into the oven and bake for approximately 10 minutes until thoroughly baked.

5. Remove from heat and set donuts onto a wire rack to cool. Add in the cream cheese (whipped) and liquid stevia in a small bowl, whisk until smooth.

6. Frost donuts using the frosting and serve with a sprinkle of cinnamon (ground) over the top.

Nutrition: Calories 95 Fats 0.3 g

Carbohydrates 9.3 g Protein 12.5 g

105. Coconut Fat Bombs

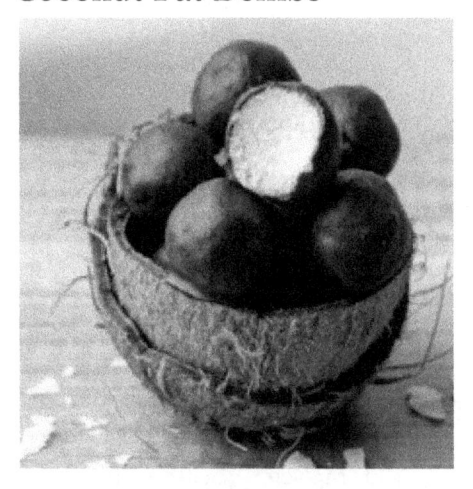

Preparation Time: 2 minutes

Cooking Time: 10 minutes

Servings: 4

Level of difficulty: Easy

Category: Green

Ingredients:

- 2/3 cup coconut oil, melted
- 1 (14 oz.) can coconut milk
- 18 drops stevia liquid
- 1 cup unsweetened coconut flakes

Directions:

Mix the coconut oil with the milk and stevia to combine. Stir in the coconut flakes until well distributed. Pour into silicone muffin molds and freeze for 1 hour to harden.

Nutrition: Calories: 214 Fat: 19 g

Carbohydrates: 2 g Protein: 4 g

106. Easy One-Pot Vegan Marinara

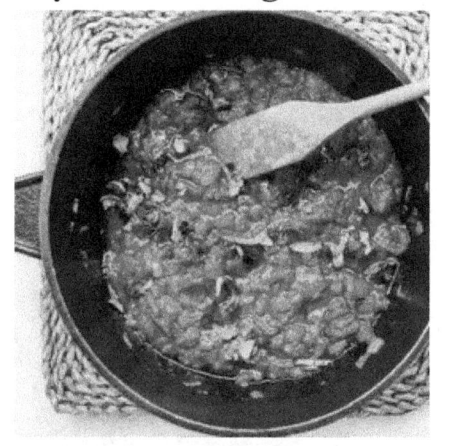

Preparation Time: 5 minutes

Cooking Time: 15 minutes

Servings: 2

Level of difficulty: Easy

Category: Green

Ingredients:

- 1 cup of water
- 1 cup tomato paste

- 2 tablespoons maple syrup
- 1 teaspoon dried oregano
- 1 teaspoon dried thyme
- 1 teaspoon garlic powder
- 1 teaspoon onion powder
- 1/2 teaspoon dried basil
- 1/4 teaspoon red pepper flakes

Directions:

1. Boil the 1 cup of water in your medium saucepan over high heat.
2. Reduce the heat to low, and whisk in the tomato paste, maple syrup, oregano, thyme, garlic powder, onion powder, basil, and red pepper flakes.
3. Cover and simmer for 10 minutes, stirring occasionally. Serve warm.

Nutrition: Calories: 79 Fat: 0g

Carbohydrates: 17 g Protein: 3 g

107. Sunflower Parmesan Cheese

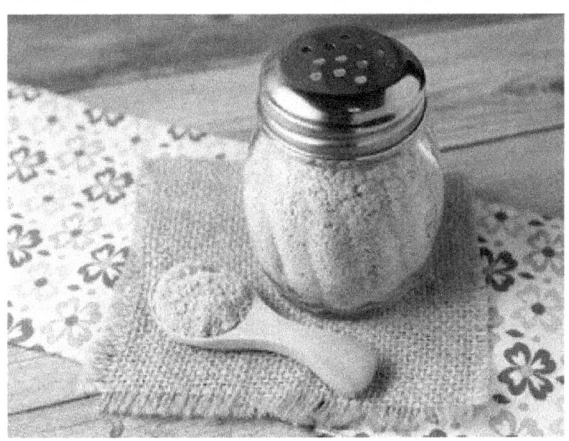

Preparation Time: 5 minutes

Cooking Time: 0 minutes

Servings: 1

Level of difficulty: Easy

Category: Healthy Fat

Ingredients:

- 1/2 cup sunflower seeds
- 2 tablespoons nutritional yeast
- 1/2 teaspoon garlic powder

Directions:

1. Process the sunflower seeds, nutritional yeast, and garlic powder in a food processor or blender.
2. Process it on low for 30 to 45 seconds, or until the sunflower seeds have been broken down to the size of coarse sea salt.
3. Store in a secure container in the refrigerator for up to 2 months.

Nutrition:

Calories: 121

Fat: 4 g

Carbohydrates: 3 g

Protein: 3 g

108. Spicy Zucchini Slices

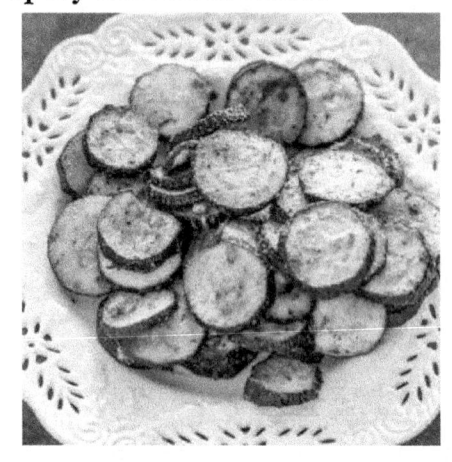

Preparation Time: 10 minutes

Cooking Time: 6 minutes

Servings: 2

Level of difficulty: Easy

Category: Green

Ingredients:

- 1 teaspoon cornstarch
- 1 zucchini
- ½ teaspoon chili flakes
- 1 tablespoon flour
- 1 egg
- ¼ teaspoon salt

Directions:

1. Slice the zucchini and sprinkle with the chili flakes and salt. Whisk the egg into the bowl. Dip the zucchini slices into the whisked egg.
2. Combine cornstarch with the flour. Stir it. Coat the zucchini slices with the cornstarch mixture—Preheat the air fryer to 400 F.
3. Put the zucchini slices in the air fryer tray. Cook for 4 minutes, then flip the pieces to another side and cook for 2 minutes more. Serve the zucchini slices hot.

Nutrition:

Calories: 67

Fat: 2.4g

Carbs: 7.7g

Protein: 4.4g

109. Cheddar Portobello Mushrooms

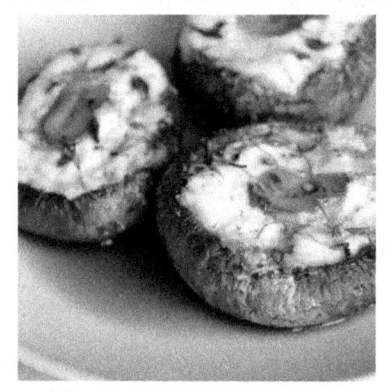

Preparation Time: 15 minutes

Cooking Time: 6 minutes

Servings: 2

Level of difficulty: Easy

Category: Green

Ingredients:

- 2 Portobello mushroom hats
- 2 slices Cheddar cheese

- ¼ cup panko breadcrumbs
- ½ teaspoon salt
- ½ teaspoon ground black pepper
- 1 egg
- 1 teaspoon oatmeal
- 2 oz. bacon, chopped cooked

Directions:

1. Whisk the egg into the bowl. Combine the ground black pepper, oatmeal, salt, and breadcrumbs in a separate bowl.
2. Dip the mushroom hats in the whisked egg. After this, coat the mushroom hats in the breadcrumb mixture.
3. Warm air fryer to 400 F. Place the mushrooms in the air fryer basket tray and cook for 3 minutes.
4. After this, put the chopped bacon and sliced cheese over the mushroom hats and cook the meal for 3 minutes. When the meal is cooked – let it chill gently.

Nutrition:

Calories: 376

Fat: 24.1g

Carbs: 14.6g

Protein: 25.2g

110. Salty Lemon Artichokes

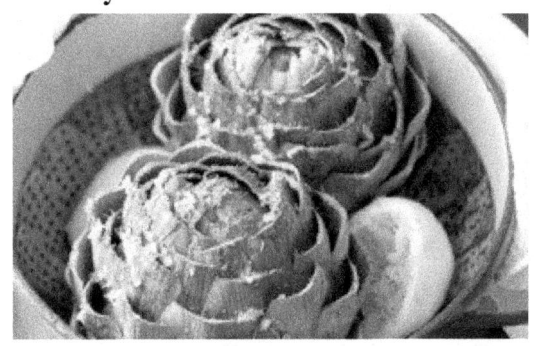

Preparation Time: 15 minutes

Cooking Time: 45 minutes

Servings: 2

Level of difficulty: Easy

Category: Green

Ingredients:

- 1 lemon
- 2 artichokes
- 1 teaspoon kosher salt
- 1 garlic head
- 2 teaspoons olive oil

Directions:

1. Cut off the edges of the artichokes. Cut the lemon into halves. Peel the garlic head and chop the garlic cloves roughly.
2. Then place the chopped garlic in the artichokes. Sprinkle the artichokes with olive oil and kosher salt. Then squeeze the lemon juice into the artichokes. Wrap the artichokes in the foil.

3. Preheat the air fryer to 330 F. Place the wrapped artichokes in the air fryer and cook for 45 minutes. When the artichokes are cooked – discard the foil and serve.

Nutrition: Calories: 133 Fat: 5g

Carbs: 21.7g Protein: 6g

111. Cheddar Potato Gratin

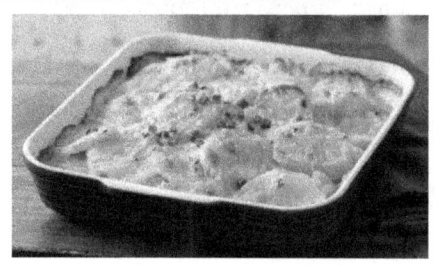

Preparation Time: 15 minutes

Cooking Time: 20 minutes

Servings: 2

Level of difficulty: Easy

Category: Green

Ingredients:

- 2 potatoes, thinly sliced
- 1/3 cup half and half
- 1 tablespoon oatmeal flour
- ¼ teaspoon ground black pepper
- 1 egg - 2 oz. Cheddar cheese

Directions:

1. Preheat the air fryer to 365 F. Put the potato slices in the air fryer and cook them for 10 minutes.

2. Meanwhile, combine the half and half, oatmeal flour, and ground black pepper. Crack the egg into the liquid and whisk it carefully—Shred Cheddar cheese.

3. When the potato is cooked – take 2 ramekins and place the potatoes on them. Pour the half and half mixture.

4. Sprinkle the gratin with shredded Cheddar cheese. Cook the gratin for 10 minutes at 360 F. Serve the meal immediately.

Nutrition: Calories: 353 Fat: 16.6g

Carbs: 37.2g Protein: 15g

112. Parmesan Sweet Potato Casserole

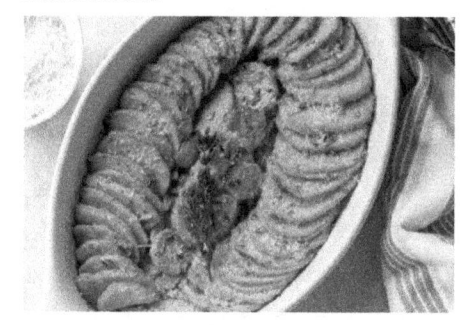

Preparation Time: 15 minutes

Cooking Time: 35 minutes

Servings: 2

Level of difficulty: Easy

Category: Green

Ingredients:

- 2 sweet potatoes, peeled, chopped
- ½ yellow onion, sliced

- ½ cup cream
- ¼ cup spinach, chopped
- 2 oz. Parmesan cheese, shredded
- ½ teaspoon salt
- 1 tomato, chopped
- 1 teaspoon olive oil

Directions:

1. Spray the air fryer tray with the olive oil. Then place on the layer of the chopped sweet potato. Add the layer of the sliced onion.
2. After this, sprinkle the sliced onion with the chopped spinach and tomatoes. Sprinkle the casserole with salt and shredded cheese. Pour cream.
3. Preheat the air fryer to 390 F. Cover the air fryer tray with the foil. Cook the casserole for 35 minutes. When the casserole is cooked – serve it.

Nutrition: Calories: 93 Fat: 1.8g

Carbs: 20.3g Protein: 1.8g

113. Asparagus & Parmesan

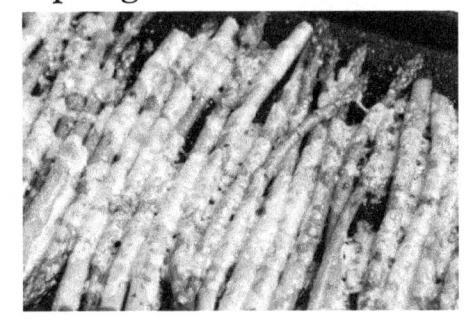

Preparation Time: 10 minutes

Cooking Time: 6 minutes

Servings: 2

Level of difficulty: Easy

Category: Green

Ingredients:

- 1 teaspoon sesame oil
- 11 oz. asparagus
- 1 teaspoon chicken stock
- ½ teaspoon ground white pepper
- 3 oz. Parmesan

Directions:

1. Wash the asparagus and chop it roughly. Sprinkle the chopped asparagus with the chicken stock and ground white pepper.
2. Then sprinkle the vegetables with the sesame oil and shake them. Place the asparagus in the air fryer basket— Cook the vegetables for 4 minutes at 400 F.
3. Meanwhile, shred Parmesan cheese. When the time is over – shake the asparagus gently and sprinkle with the shredded cheese.
4. Cook the asparagus for 2 minutes more at 400 F. After this, transfer the cooked asparagus to the serving plates. Serve and taste it!

Nutrition: Calories: 189 Fat: 11.6g

Carbs: 7.9g Protein: 17.2g

CHAPTER 8:

Seafood

114. Shrimp Spring Rolls

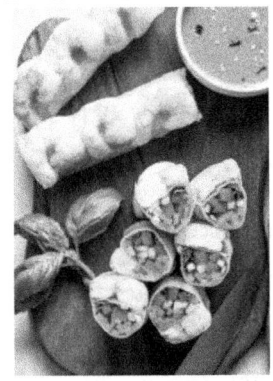

Preparation time: 10 minutes

Cooking time: 25 minutes

Servings: 4

Level of difficulty: Easy

Category: Leanest

Ingredients:

- ½ cup deveined raw shrimp, chopped & peeled
- 2 and 1/2 tbsp olive oil
- 1 cup matchstick carrots
- 1 cup slices of red bell pepper
- 1/4 teaspoon red pepper, crushed
- 3/4 cup slices of snow peas
- 2 cups shredded cabbage
- 1 tablespoon lime juice
- 1/2 cup sweet chili sauce
- 2 teaspoons fish sauce
- 8 spring roll (wrappers)

Directions:

1. In a skillet, add one and a half tbsp of olive until smoking lightly. Stir in bell pepper, cabbage, carrots, and cook for two minutes. Turn off the heat, take out in a dish and cool for five minutes.
2. In a bowl, add shrimp, lime juice, cabbage mixture, crushed red pepper, fish sauce, and snow peas. Mix well.
3. Lay spring roll wrappers on a plate. Add 1/4 cup of filling in the middle of each wrapper. Fold tightly with water. Brush the olive oil over folded rolls.
4. Put spring rolls in the air fryer basket and cook for 6 to 7 minutes at 390°F until light brown and crispy. You may serve with sweet chili sauce.

Nutrition: Calories 180 Fat 9g

Protein 17g Carbohydrate 9g

115. Scallops with Tomato Cream Sauce

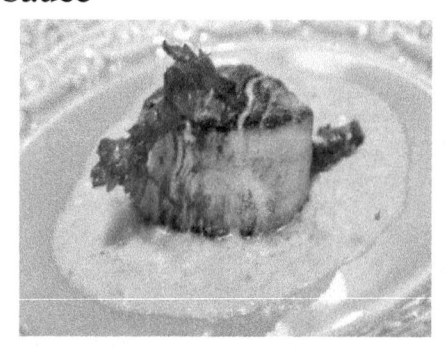

Preparation time: 5 minutes

Cooking time: 10 minutes

Servings: 2

Level of difficulty: Normal

Category: Leanest

Ingredients:

- 8 sea scallops, jumbo
- 1 tbsp tomato paste
- 1 tbsp chopped fresh basil
- 3/4 cup of low-fat whipping cream
- ½ tsp kosher salt
- ½ tsp ground freshly black pepper
- 1 tsp minced garlic
- ½ cup frozen spinach, thawed
- oil spray

Directions:

1. Take a seven-inch pan(heatproof) and add spinach in a single layer at the bottom. Rub olive oil on both sides of scallops, season with kosher salt and pepper.
2. Place the seasoned scallops on top of the spinach. Put the pan in the air fryer and cook for ten minutes at 350F, until scallops are cooked thoroughly and internal temperature reaches 135F. Serve immediately.

Nutrition:

Calories: 259

Carbohydrates: 6g

Protein: 19g

Fat: 13g

116. Sriracha & Honey Tossed Calamari

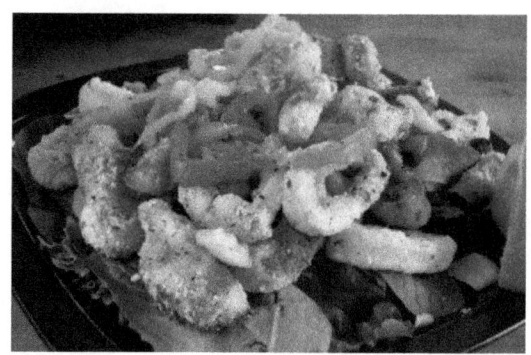

Preparation time: 10 minutes

Cooking time: 20 minutes

Servings: 2

Level of difficulty: Normal

Category: Leaner

Ingredients:

- 1 cup club soda

- 1-2 tbsp sriracha
- 2 cups calamari tubes
- 1 cup flour
- pinches of salt
- ground black pepper
- red pepper flakes
- red pepper
- 1/2 cup honey

Directions:

1. Cut the calamari tubes into rings. Submerge them with club soda. Let it rest for ten minutes. Put freshly ground black pepper, flour, red pepper, kosher salt in a bowl, and mix well.
2. Drain the calamari and pat dry with a paper towel. Coat the calamari well in the flour mix and set aside. Spray oil in the air fryer basket and put calamari in one single layer.
3. Cook at 375 for 11 minutes. Toss the rings twice while cooking. Meanwhile, to make sauce honey, red pepper flakes, and sriracha in a bowl, well.
4. Take calamari out from the basket, mix with sauce cook for another two minutes more. Serve with salad green.

Nutrition:

Cal 252 Fat: 38g

Carbs: 3.1g Protein: 41g

117. Southern Style Catfish with Green Beans

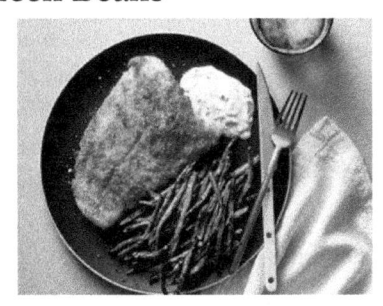

Preparation time: 10 minutes

Cooking time: 20 minutes

Servings: 2

Level of difficulty: Normal

Category: Leanest

Ingredients:

- 2 pieces catfish fillets
- ½ cup green beans, trimmed
- 2 tsp honey
- ground black pepper
- salt - ½ crushed red pepper
- ¼ cup flour
- 1 egg, lightly beaten
- 3/4 teaspoon dill pickle relish
- ½ tsp apple cider vinegar
- 1/3 cup whole-wheat breadcrumbs
- 2 tablespoons mayonnaise
- dill
- lemon wedges

Directions:

1. In a bowl, add green beans, spray them with cooking oil. Coat with crushed red pepper, 1/8 teaspoon of kosher salt, and half tsp of honey and cook in the air fryer at 400 F until soft and browned, for 12 minutes. Take out from fryer and cover with aluminum foil.

2. In the meantime, coat catfish in flour. Then dip in egg to coat, then in breadcrumbs. Place fish in an air fryer basket and spray with cooking oil.

3. Cook for 8 minutes, at 400°F, until cooked through and golden brown. Sprinkle with pepper and salt. In the meantime, mix vinegar, dill, relish, mayonnaise, and honey in a bowl. Serve the sauce with fish and green beans.

Nutrition: Cal 243 Fat 18 g

Carbs 18 g Protein 33 g

118. Roasted Salmon with Fennel Salad

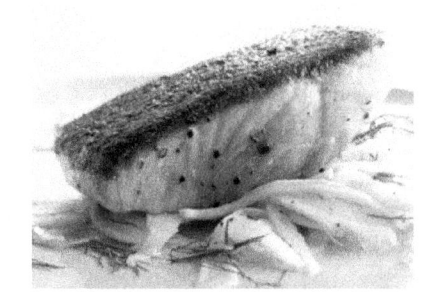

Preparation time: 15 minutes

Cooking time: 10 minutes

Servings: 4

Level of difficulty: Normal

Category: Lean

Ingredients:

- 4 salmon fillets, skinless and center-cut
- 1 teaspoon lemon juice, fresh
- 2 teaspoons parsley, chopped
- 1 teaspoon salt, divided
- 2 tablespoons olive oil
- 1 teaspoon chopped thyme
- 4 cups fennel heads, thinly sliced
- 1 clove of minced garlic
- 2 tablespoons fresh dill, chopped
- 2 tablespoons orange juice, fresh
- 2/3 cup Greek yogurt, reduced-fat

Directions:

1. Mix half a teaspoon of salt, parsley, and thyme in a bowl. Rub oil over salmon, and sprinkle with thyme mixture.

2. Put salmon fillets in the air fryer basket, cook for ten minutes at 350°F. In the meantime, mix garlic, fennel, orange juice, yogurt, half tsp of salt, dill, lemon juice in a bowl. Serve with fennel salad.

Nutrition: Calories 364 Fat 30g

Protein 38g Carbohydrate 9g

119. Catfish with Cajun Seasoning

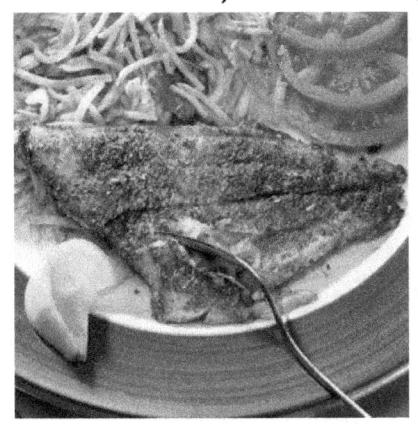

Preparation time: 5 minutes

Cooking time: 20 minutes

Servings: 4

Level of difficulty: Easy

Category: Leanest

Ingredients:

- 3 teaspoons Cajun seasoning
- 3/4 cup Cornmeal
- 4 catfish fillets

Directions:

1. Put Cajun seasoning and cornmeal in a zip lock bag. Wash and pat dry the catfish fillets. Add them to the zip lock bag.
2. Coat well the fillets with seasoning. Put catfish fillets in the air fryer. And cook within 15 minutes at 390 F, turn fillets halfway through.
3. To get a golden color on the fillets, cook for more 5 minutes. Serve with lemon wedges and spicy tartar sauce.

Nutrition:

Cal 324

Fat: 13.9g

Carbohydrates: 15.6g

Protein: 26.3g

120. Sushi Roll

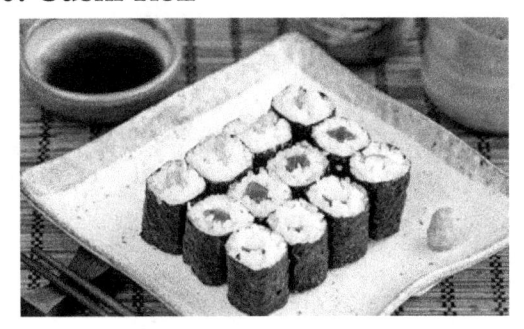

Preparation time: 1 hour & 30 minutes

Cooking time: 10 minutes

Servings: 3

Level of difficulty: Normal

Category: Lean

Ingredients:

For the Kale Salad:

- ½ tsp rice vinegar
- 1 and 1/2 cups chopped kale
- 1/8 teaspoon garlic powder
- 1 tablespoon sesame seeds
- 3/4 teaspoon toasted sesame oil
- 1/4 teaspoon ground ginger
- 3/4 teaspoon

Soy sauce:

- sushi rolls
- 1/2 avocado, sliced
- cooked sushi rice cooled
- ½ cup whole wheat breadcrumbs
- 3 sheets of sushi

Directions:

1. In a bowl, add vinegar, garlic powder, kale, soy sauce, sesame oil, and ground ginger. With your hands, mix with sesame seeds and set them aside.
2. Lay a sheet of sushi on a flat surface. With damp fingertips, add a tablespoon of rice, and spread it on the sheet. Cover the sheet with rice leaving a half-inch space at one end.
3. Add kale salad with avocado slices. Roll up the sushi, use water if needed. Add the breadcrumbs to a bowl. Coat the sushi roll with Sriracha Mayo, then in breadcrumbs.
4. Add the rolls to the air fryer. Cook for ten minutes at 390 F, shake the basket halfway through. Take out from the fryer, and let them cool, then cut with a sharp knife. Serve with soy sauce.

Nutrition:

Calories: 369

Fat: 13.9g

Carbohydrates: 15g

Protein: 26.3g

121. Garlic-Lime Shrimp Kebabs

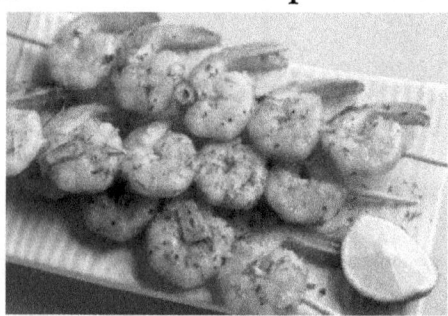

Preparation time: 5 minutes

Cooking time: 18 minutes

Servings: 2

Level of difficulty: Easy

Category: Leanest

Ingredients:

- 1 lime - 1 cup raw shrimp
- 1/8 tsp Salt
- 1 clove of garlic
- Freshly ground black pepper

Directions:

1. In water, let wooden skewers soak for 20 minutes. Let the Air fryer preheat to 350F. In a bowl, mix shrimp, minced garlic, lime juice, kosher salt, and pepper. Add shrimp on skewers.
2. Place skewers in the air fryer, and cook for 8 minutes. Turn halfway over. Top with cilantro and your favorite dip.

Nutrition: Calories: 76 Carbohydrates: 4g

Protein: 13g Fat 9 g

122. Fish Finger Sandwich

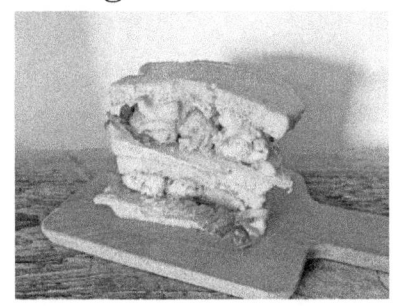

Preparation time: 10 minutes

Cooking time: 20 minutes

Servings: 3

Category: Leanest

Level of difficulty: Normal

Ingredients:

- 1 tbsp Greek yogurt
- 4 cod fillets, without skin
- 2 tbsp flour
- 5 tbsp whole-wheat breadcrumbs
- kosher salt and pepper, to taste
- 10-12 capers
- ¾ cup frozen peas
- lemon juice

Directions:

1. Let the air fryer preheat. Sprinkle kosher salt and pepper on the cod fillets, and coat in flour, then in breadcrumbs
2. Spray the fryer basket with oil. Put the cod fillets in the basket. Cook for 15 minutes at 200 C.
3. In the meantime, cook the peas in boiling water for a few minutes. Take out from the water and blend with Greek yogurt, lemon juice, and capers until well combined. On a bun, add cooked fish with pea puree. Add lettuce and tomato.

Nutrition:

Cal 240

Fat: 12g

Carbs: 7g

Protein: 20g

123. Healthy Tuna Patties

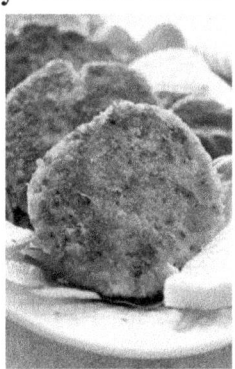

Preparation time: 15 minutes

Cooking time: 10 minutes

Servings: 10

Level of difficulty: Normal

Category: Leanest

Ingredients:

- ½ cup whole wheat breadcrumbs
- 4 cups fresh tuna, diced

- lemon zest
- 1 tbsp lemon juice
- 1 egg
- 3 tbsp grated parmesan cheese
- 1 chopped stalk celery
- ½ tsp garlic powder
- ½ tsp dried herbs
- 3 tbsp minced onion
- salt, to taste
- freshly ground black pepper

Directions:

1. In a bowl, add lemon zest, bread crumbs, salt, pepper, celery, eggs, dried herbs, lemon juice, garlic powder, parmesan cheese, and onion. Mix everything.
2. Then add in tuna gently. Shape into patties, and if the mixture is too loose, cool in the refrigerator. Add air fryer baking paper in the air fryer basket. Spray the baking paper with cooking spray.
3. Spray the patties with oil—Cook for ten minutes at 360°F. Turn the patties halfway over. Serve with lemon slices and microgreens.

Nutrition:

Cal 214 Fat: 15g

Carbs: 6g

Protein: 22g

124. Crab Cakes

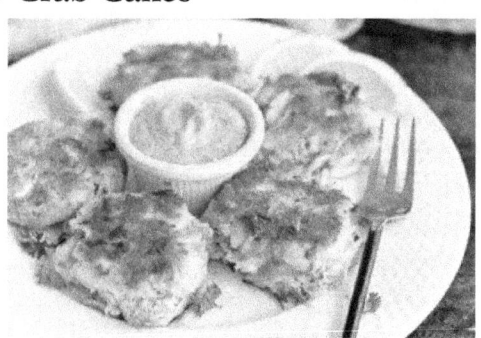

Preparation time: 10 minutes

Cooking time: 20 minutes

Servings: 6

Level of difficulty: Normal

Category: Leanest

Ingredients:

- 4 cups of crab meat
- 2 eggs
- ¼ cup whole wheat bread crumbs
- 2 tbsp mayonnaise
- 1 tsp Worcestershire sauce
- 1 ½ tsp old bay seasoning
- 1 tsp Dijon mustard
- freshly ground black pepper to taste
- ¼ cup green onion, chopped

Directions:

1. In a bowl, add Dijon mustard, Old Bay, eggs, Worcestershire, and mayonnaise mix it well. Then add in the chopped green onion and mix.

2. Fold in the crab meat to mayonnaise mix. Then add breadcrumbs, not to over mix. Chill the mixture in the refrigerator for at least 60 minutes. Then shape into patties.

3. Let the air-fryer preheat to 350F. Cook for 10 minutes. Flip the patties halfway through. Serve with lemon wedges.

Nutrition:

Cal 218 Fat: 13 g

Carbs: 5.6 g Protein: 16.7g

125. Breaded Air Fried Shrimp with Bang-Bang Sauce

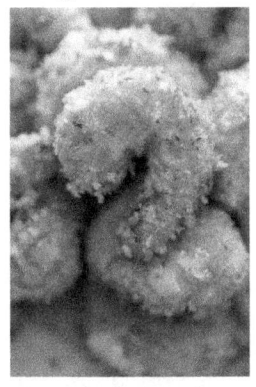

Preparation time: 10 minutes

Cooking time: 20 minutes

Servings: 4

Level of difficulty: Normal

Category: Leanest

Ingredients:

- 3/4 cup whole wheat bread crumbs
- 4 cups raw shrimp, deveined, peeled
- 1 tsp ½ cup flour
- 1 tsp paprika
- chicken seasoning, to taste
- 2 tbsp. of one egg white
- kosher salt and pepper to taste

Bang-Bang Sauce:

- ¼ cup sweet chili sauce
- 1/3 cup plain Greek yogurt
- 2 tbsp sriracha

Directions:

1. Let the Air Fryer preheat to 400 degrees. Add the seasonings to shrimp and coat well. In three separate bowls, add flour, bread crumbs, and egg whites.

2. First coat the shrimp in flour, dab lightly in egg whites, then in the bread crumbs. With cooking oil, spray the shrimp.

3. Place the shrimps in an air fryer, cook for four minutes, turn the shrimp over, and cook for another four minutes. In a small bowl, mix all the bang-bang ingredients. Serve with micro green and bang-bang sauce.

Nutrition:

Calories 229

Fat 10g

Carbohydrates 13g

Protein 22g

126. Crispy Fish Sandwich

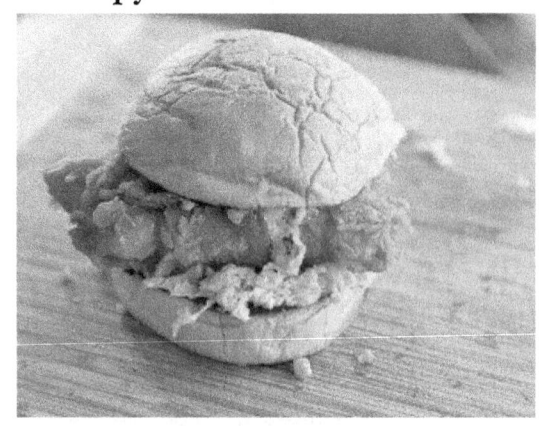

Preparation time: 15 minutes

Cooking time: 10 minutes

Servings: 2

Level of difficulty: Normal

Category: Leanest

Ingredients:

- 2 fillets cod
- 2 tbsp all-purpose flour
- ¼ tsp pepper
- 1 tbsp lemon juice
- ¼ tsp salt
- ½ tsp garlic powder
- 1 egg
- ½ tbsp mayo
- ½ cup whole wheat bread crumbs

Directions:

1. In a bowl, add salt, flour, pepper, and garlic powder. In a separate bowl, add lemon juice, mayo, and egg. In another bowl, add the breadcrumbs.
2. Coat the fish in flour, then in egg, then in breadcrumbs. With cooking oil, spray the basket and put the fish in the basket.
3. Also, spray the fish with cooking oil. Cook at 400 F for ten minutes. This fish is soft, be careful if you flip.

Nutrition:

Cal 218

Carbs:7g

Fat:12g

Protein: 22g

127. Shrimp Egg Rolls

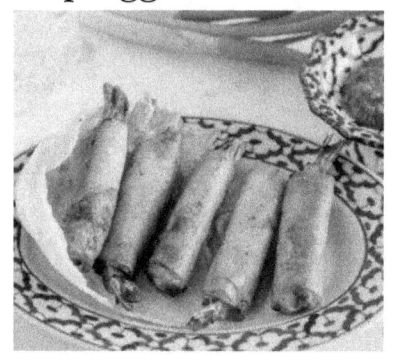

Preparation time: 20 minutes

Cooking time: 20 minutes

Servings: 6

Level of difficulty: Normal

Category: Leanest

Ingredients:

- 2-3 cloves of minced garlic

- 12-14 egg roll wrappers
- 2-3 cloves of minced garlic
- 4 cups raw shrimp, roughly chopped, peeled, and deveined
- 3 cups coleslaw mix
- 1 ½ tsp sesame oil
- 1 tbsp soy sauce
- 1 tsp fish sauce
- salt, pepper to taste
- ½ tsp grated ginger
- 2 green onions, chopped
- 1 cup water

Directions:

1. In a skillet, add shrimp with garlic, kosher salt, and pepper, spray with cooking oil and sauté until shrimp is pink. Set it aside.
2. In a bowl, add coleslaw mix, cooked shrimp, green onions, fish sauce, soy sauce, sesame oil, and ginger. Mix well.
3. Add two tbsp of filling to each wrapper, seal tightly with water. With cooking oil, spray the air fryer basket. Put the egg rolls in a single layer in the basket. Spray with cooking oil.
4. Cook for 7 minutes at 400 degrees. Flip the rolls, then cook for 5 minutes more. Serve with a microgreen salad.

Nutrition:

Calories 228

Fat 11g

Carbs 11g

Protein 20g

CHAPTER 9:

Vegetables Dishes

128. Arugula Lentil Salad

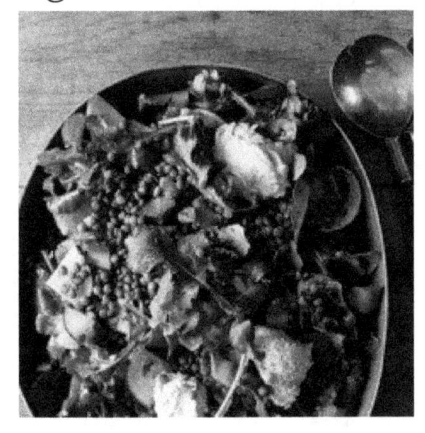

Preparation time: 5 minutes

Cooking time: 7 minutes

Servings: 2

Level of difficulty: Easy

Category: Green

Ingredients:

- 1-2 tbsp. balsamic vinegar
- ¾ cups cashews
- 1 handful arugula/rocket
- 1 cup brown lentils, cooked
- slices bread, whole wheat
- 5-6 sun-dried tomatoes in oil
- 1 chili / jalapeño
- 1 tbsp. olive oil
- 1 onion
- salt and pepper to taste

Optional:

- 1 tbsp. honey
- 1 small handful of raisins

Directions:

1. Toast the cashews in a pan over low heat for about 3 to 4 minutes. Then dump them into a pot of salad. Dice and fry the onion in one-third of the olive oil over low heat for around 3 minutes.

2. In the meantime, cut your chili / jalapeño and dried tomatoes. In the grill, add them and fry for the next 1-2 minutes.

3. Slice the bread into large croutons. Shift the mixture of onions into a large container. Put the rest of the oil in your pan and cook the sliced bread until it's crispy with salt and pepper seasoning.

4. Now clean the arugula and put it in the bowl. Bring in the lentils, too,

and blend everything over. Use salt, pepper, and balsamic vinegar to season. With the croutons, eat. Super delicious!

Nutrition:

Calories: 270 Carbs: 27g

Fat: 15g Protein: 12g

129. Tomato Avocado Toast

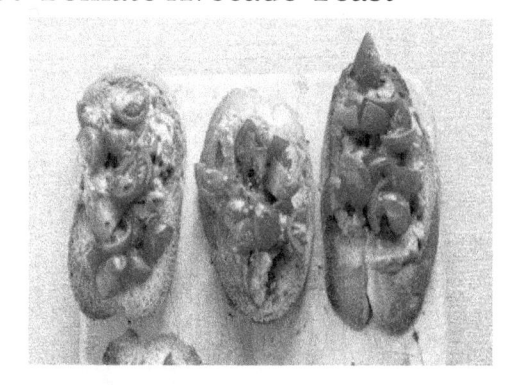

Preparation time: 5 minutes

Cooking time: 5 minutes

Servings: 1 toast

Level of difficulty: Easy

Category: Green

Ingredients:

- 1 slice bread (ideally whole grain)
- ½ medium avocado
- 1 tbsp. lemon juice
- 1 tbsp. olive oil
- salt and pepper to taste
- cherry tomatoes

Directions:

1. Split in half your cherry tomatoes. Dump them in a pan and let them cook until tender (about 5 minutes) with olive oil.
2. In the meantime, mash and add some lemon with your avocado. Put it all together now, and season with salt and pepper. Perfect.

Nutrition:

Calories: 285 Carbs: 25g

Fat: 16g Protein: 11g

130. Classic Tofu Salad

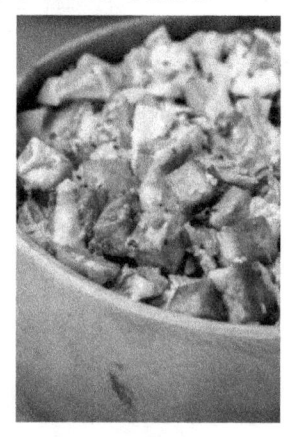

Preparation time: 5 minutes

Cooking time: 15 minutes

Servings: 2

Level of difficulty: Normal

Category: Green

Ingredients:

- 8 oz pineapple

- 1 handful spinach
- ½ bunch radishes
- ½ medium cucumber
- 1 cup bean sprouts
- 14 oz. firm tofu (ideally get fresh tofu from the supermarket)

For the dressing:

- 1 tbsp. olive oil
- salt and pepper to taste
- 1 small handful of peanuts
- ½ chili pepper (e.g., jalapeño)
- ½ lime (juiced; lemon also works)
- 1 tbsp. sriracha (or equivalent)
- 1 tbsp. maple syrup

Directions:

1. Squeeze out some of the tofu block's excess moisture, and split it (about one square centimeter) into tiny cubes. Heat some oil in a pan over low to medium heat and add it to your tofu.
2. Fry until golden brown for approximately 15 minutes. Rinse the vegetables! Chop the radishes. Lengthwise, slice the cucumber in half, scrape the seeds with a big spoon, and cut what's left.
3. Also, cut the pineapple into smaller pieces. Put all together with the bean sprouts and spinach into a dish.
4. For the dressing, put the sugar, olive oil, sriracha, lime juice, salt, and pepper together and toss in the salad.
5. Get the pieces of tofu and put them in a separate bowl. Mix them to every serving of salad. Cut the chili and slightly crush or chop the peanuts for garnish as well. When served, dust them over the salad. Enjoy!

Nutrition:

Calories: 84

Carbs: 3g

Fat: 4g

Protein: 9g

131. Moroccan Couscous Salad

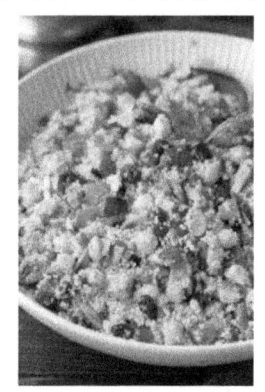

Preparation time: 15 minutes

Cooking time: 0 minutes

Servings: 6

Level of difficulty: Normal

Category: Green

Ingredients:

- 2 tbsp. olive oil

- fig, fresh
- ½ orange's zest
- orange
- 1 medium zucchini
- 1 pomegranate
- 1 tbsp. ginger powder, chopped
- 1 tbsp. cumin
- 1 tbsp. paprika powder
- 1 bell pepper, red
- ½ cup parsley, fresh
- 1 tbsp. salt
- salt and pepper to taste
- 1 cup of water
- ¼ cup raisins
- 1 cup instant couscous

Optional:
1. bunch radish (thinly sliced)

Directions:
1. Put water in a wide serving bowl and apply it to the couscous. Cover a tea towel or lid with the couscous and leave for 5 minutes.
2. Gently loosen the couscous with a fork and add the cumin, ginger, olive oil, and paprika powder. You want it dry and cool, no big clumps.
3. Wash the cherry, rub the zest. Peel and chop the orange and, along with the zest, add it to the salad.
4. Deseed and apply the seeds to the pomegranate. Finely cut the zucchini and thinly slice the red pepper, then put it in the salad.
5. Cut it up and add it to the salad if you've managed to find a fig. Clean the parsley and any other optional herbs, chop them, and then return them to the salad again. Give a decent toss to it. Serve.

Nutrition:Calories: 206 Carbs: 34g

Fat: 5g Protein: 7g

132. Eggplant Curry

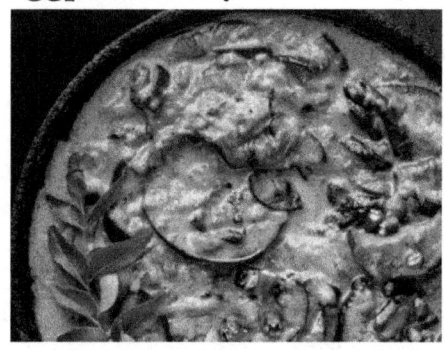

Preparation time: 15 minutes

Cooking time: 30 minutes

Servings: 2

Level of difficulty: Normal

Category: Green

Ingredients:
- ½ tbsp. pepper

- ½ cups of coconut milk
- 1 tin tomatoes, chopped roughly
- 1 tbsp. ground coriander
- 1 tbsp. turmeric
- 1 tbsp. gram masala powder or curry powder
- 1 clove garlic
- 1 red onion
- 1 tbsp olive oil
- ½ tbsp salt
- 1 aborigine (medium)

Optional:

- 1-2 tbsp. sugar or mango chutney

Directions:

1. Cook as per packet directions when using rice. Break your aubergine into tiny cubes. Fry with olive oil in a wide pan over high heat for 3-4 minutes. Mix well enough that it won't smoke.
2. Meanwhile, chop the onion, and put it in as well. Put it back to medium heat and cook for 5-6 minutes. Crush the garlic or dice it.
3. Garlic, curry powder, turmeric, and ground cilantro should be mixed in. Cook, stirring well, for the next 3-4 minutes. Add in the sliced tomatoes and coconut milk. Add salt.
4. Boil for 15 minutes, roughly. The coconut milk gets thicker, so when it is at the right consistency for you, stop cooking.
5. If you like it a little sweeter, stir in the honey or mango chutney. Serve with salt plus pepper according to taste.

Nutrition:

Calories: 200

Carbs: 18g

Fat: 0g

Protein: 0g

133. Asian Cabbage Rice

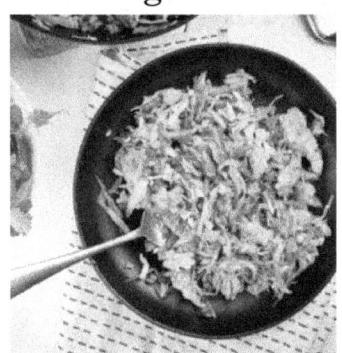

Preparation time: 15 minutes

Cooking time: 7 minutes

Servings: 2

Level of difficulty: Easy

Category: Green

Ingredients:

- 1-2 fresh lime slice
- 1/2 cup water
- 1 tbsp Thai Seasoning

- 4 cups cabbage, minced into a rice-like texture
- fresh cilantro & green onion (optional)

Directions:

1. Mince the cabbage into perfect texture-like rice. Sauté the cabbage and spices in the lime juice in water for 1-2 minutes over medium heat.
2. Squeeze 1-2 lime slices over the cabbage and simmer until tender for another 3-5 minutes, stirring periodically and adding water if needed. Remove from heat and blend just before serving with fresh, minced cilantro.

Nutrition:

Calories: 170 Carbs: 0g

Fat: 13g Protein: 3g

134. African Peanut Soup

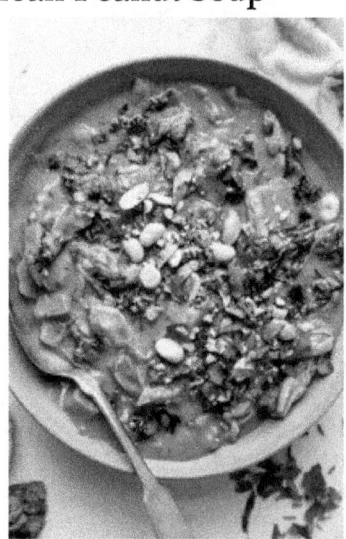

Preparation time: 15 minutes

Cooking time: 10 minutes

Servings: 3

Level of difficulty: Easy

Category: Green

Ingredients:

- 1 cup brown rice (uncooked)
- A few dashes of hot sauce
- 1 tbsp. soy sauce
- 1 clove garlic
- 1 small carrot
- 1 tbsp. tomato paste
- handful of peanuts
- 3-4 tbsp. peanut butter
- ½ medium courgette (zucchini)
- ½ red onion
- cups vegetable broth
- 1 ginger, fresh or ½ tbsp. powdered ginger

Directions:

1. Prepare the brown rice. Put to the boil 700ml of vegetable broth. Split the cabbage, carrot, and courgette and add them to the broth. Garlic and ginger are also added to the broth.
2. Put in the peanuts. Add some peanut butter and tomato paste to your mixture. Add some soy sauce last but

ensure it's not still too salty. Let the rice boil until it is done. Serve in a pot, eat it instantly.

Nutrition:

Calories: 130

Carbs: 13g

Fat: 7g

Protein: 4g

135. Sweet Potato Soup

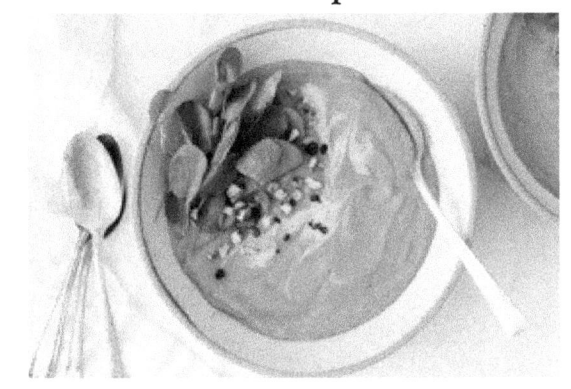

Preparation time: 10 minutes

Cooking time: 20 minutes

Servings: 4

Level of difficulty: Normal

Category: Green

Ingredients:

- 2 tbsp. olive oil
- 1 medium onion
- bell pepper, red
- 2 cloves garlic
- 1 tbsp. cinnamon
- 1 ginger, fresh, or 1 tbsp. dried ginger
- 2 cups vegetable broth
- 1 tbsp peanut butter
- ½ tbsp. cayenne pepper
- ½ cup tomato puree
- 2 ½ cups large sweet potato, chopped
- 1 tbsp. soy sauce (low sodium if necessary)
- salt and pepper to taste
- 1 tbsp. vinegar or lemon juice
- 2 tbsp. maple syrup
- peanuts (to garnish)
- ½ lime (juiced)
- ¼ cup cilantro/coriander, fresh

Directions:

1. Cut the onions and dump them into the oil in a pot on low to moderate heat. For around 5 minutes, let the onion cook steadily; it should begin to turn transparent.

2. Peel and then slice the sweet potatoes into chunks. Cut the garlic, bell pepper, and ginger and put them into the bowl. Add them now if you're using dried herbs.

3. Also, put in cinnamon and cayenne pepper. Cook and add the soy sauce, peanut butter, vinegar, and tomato

for the next two minutes. Stir well and apply a shot of broth.

4. Chuck in the sweet potatoes and most of the broth, and boil on medium heat. Add them now if you are using raw herbs. Stir regularly and after 10-15 minutes, confirm the sweet potatoes are cooked.

5. Season using salt and pepper, maple syrup, and lime juice, and allow another swirl. If you used a cinnamon stick, then throw it out now.

6. Use a hand liquidizer or offer the soup a blend on a blender if you do not have one. Garnish with peanuts, then serve with a side if desired – fresh bread is an obvious option!

Nutrition:

Calories: 110 Carbs: 23g

Fat: 1g

Protein: 2g

136. Roasted Garlic Wilted Spinach

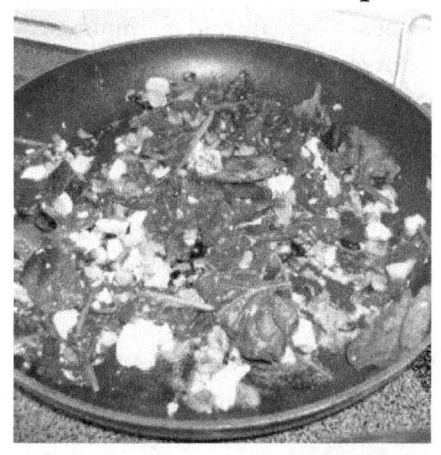

Preparation time: 15 minutes

Cooking time: 5 minutes

Servings: 2

Level of difficulty: Easy

Category: Green

Ingredients:

- 1 tbsp garlic and spring onion seasoning
- 2 cups baby spinach, rinsed
- 2 tbsp roasted garlic oil

Directions:

1. Heat-up oil over high heat in an 8-quart pot until sizzling. Apply the spinach and the seasoning and brush with a toss.

2. Put a lid on the pot and switch off the heat. Leave it for about 3 minutes to allow it to set. Take off the cover and throw the spinach once more. It's meant to be light green and wilted.

Nutrition:

Calories: 94

Carbs: 8g

Fat: 6g

Protein: 6g

137. Avocado Toast with Radish

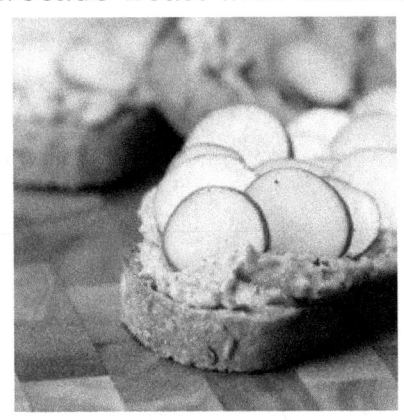

Preparation time: 15 minutes

Cooking time: 0 minutes

Servings: 1 toast

Level of difficulty: Easy

Category: Green

Ingredients:

- 1 slice bread (ideally whole grain)
- salt to taste
- 1 tbsp. lemon juice
- 1 tbsp. cilantro/coriander, fresh
- radishes
- ½ medium avocado

Directions:

1. Mash the avocado; put some salt and a splash of lemon juice. Cut the radish finely. Use cilantro as a garnish. Spicy and delicious!

Nutrition: Calories: 321 Carbs: 20g

Fat: 22g Protein: 12g

138. Baba Ganoush

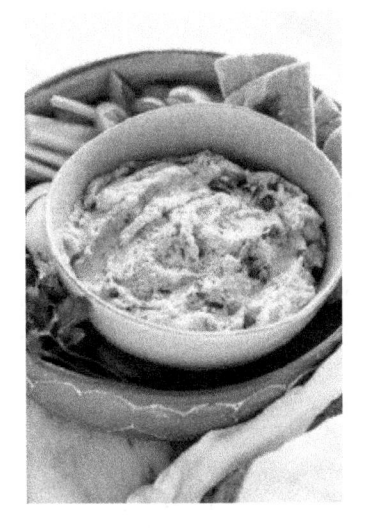

Preparation time: 15 minutes

Cooking time: 0 minutes

Servings: 8-10

Level of difficulty: Normal

Category: Green

Ingredients:

- 3 small eggplants
- salt and pepper to taste
- 1 tbsp. paprika
- 1 tbsp. olive oil (plus a splash when serving the dish)
- 1 lemon (juiced)
- 1 tbsp. tahini (or sesame paste is fine too)
- 1 cloves garlic

Optional:

- 1 tbsp. cilantro/coriander, fresh

- handful pomegranate seeds

Directions:

1. Warm your oven to 180 C. Place the eggplants on an oven tray with a drizzle of olive oil and some spices. Prick mini holes in it using a toothpick.
2. Put the cloves of garlic; no reason for them to peel. Roast before tender for about 25-30 minutes.
3. Let it cool, then slice them open and slice out the flesh. Using a beater or food blender, mix the eggplant flesh with the juice of the lemon.
4. Put in a bowl with some paprika and a dash of olive oil for garnish. You can serve as a dip with pitas, flatbread, or nachos or as a side dish with the main dish.
5. For optional, stir in the pomegranate seeds and cilantro to add an extra kick of freshness to this lovely Baba Ganoush.

Nutrition:

Calories: 349

Carbs: 5g

Fat: 29g

Protein: 12g

139. Black Bean Burgers

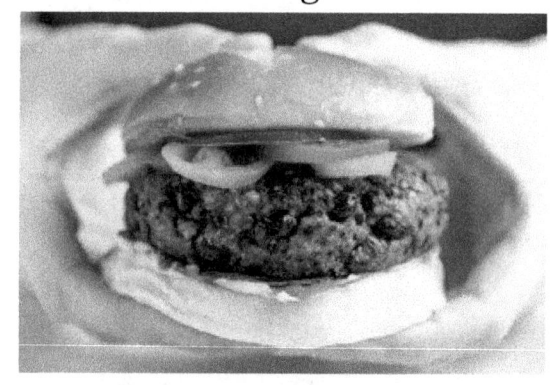

Preparation time: 15 minutes

Cooking time: 10 minutes

Servings: 8 burgers

Level of difficulty: Normal

Category: Green

Ingredients:

- ½ cup dried breadcrumbs
- ½ cup sun-dried tomatoes in oil
- 2 tbsp. olive oil
- ½ medium red onion
- 1 tbsp. paprika
- 1½ tbsp. cumin
- ½ tbsp. salt
- 1 can of black beans
- 1 Egg
- ½ cup rolled oats

Directions:

1. Wash and drain the black beans. Blend with a hand blender and place

it in a big mixing bowl. Conversely, crush the beans with a fork/masher.

2. Dice the red onion and sundried tomatoes and add them to the dish. Then add some salt, chickens, cumin, oats, paprika, olive oil, etc. Give a nice stir to it.

3. Finally, put some of the breadcrumbs until you're left with a good, firm mixture. If you don't need to use all the breadcrumbs, that's cool. Sculpt the paste into patties for burgers. If it is too sticky, wet your hands a little.

4. Fry in a pan with a little oil, or place on a grill. Cook on both sides within 5 minutes, turning occasionally. Serve whatever you fancy with your favorite burger ingredients: a bun, lettuce, tomato, cheese!

Nutrition:

Calories: 95 Carbs: 18g

Fat: 1g

Protein: 6g

140. Chickpea Flour Pancake Fennel & Olive

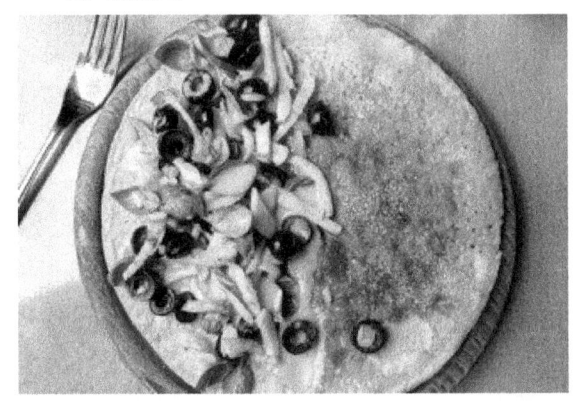

Preparation time: 5 minutes

Cooking time: 20 minutes

Servings: 2

Level of difficulty: Normal

Category: Green

Ingredients:

- 1 handful basil, fresh
- ¼ cup olives pitted
- ½ cup of water
- ½ bulbs. fennel
- 2 tbsp. olive oil
- 1 clove garlic (or garlic salt)
- ½ cup chickpea flour
- Salt and pepper to taste

For the sauce:

- Salt and pepper to taste
- 1 tbsp. maple syrup
- 1 tbsp. mustard
- 1 tbsp. olive oil
- 2 tbsp. water
- 2 tbsp. vinegar

Directions:

1. For the filling, cut the fennel into pieces. Chop the olives. Crush or very finely chop the garlic clove (if using any).

2. Take a pot, set it to low-medium heat. Sauté the fennel in a splash of olive oil (or a tbsp. or two water) for 7-8 minutes. At that point, include the olives and garlic and fry for an additional 5 minutes.

3. Take a bowl and put the chickpea flour and salt (or garlic salt) for the pancakes. Put the water while mixing the batter well with a fork. If you have a whisk, use one.

4. Place the pan over medium heat, add the olive oil and pour half the mixture into the pan. Cook for 4-5 minutes roughly. Turn, and then fry for the next 4-5 minutes. It should come out crispy when done.

5. For the sauce, blend the water, vinegar, olive oil, maple syrup, mustard, salt, and pepper in a tiny bowl.

6. When it's done, put them on a plate. Spread out the fennel-olive blend and put some fresh basil leaves on top of that. Complete your dish with a drizzle of mustard sauce.

Nutrition:

Calories: 93

Carbs: 9g

Fat: 4g

Protein: 3g

141. Colorful Tabbouleh Salad

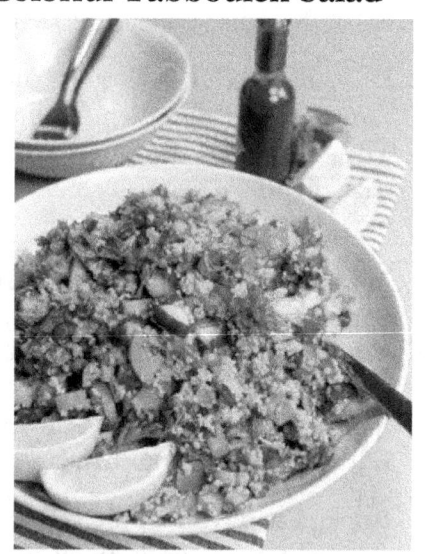

Preparation time: 15 minutes

Cooking time: 0 minutes

Servings: 4

Level of difficulty: Normal

Category: Green

Ingredients:

- 1 cup instant couscous
- salt and pepper to taste
- 4 tbsp. olive oil
- 2 1/2 tbsp. tomato paste
- 2 small tomato
- 7 sun-dried tomatoes in oil
- 2 spring onions
- 1 bunch parsley, fresh
- ½ cucumber

- 1 carrot
- 1 lemon (juiced)
- 1 1/2 cups vegetable broth (or just use water)

Optional

- 1 tbsp. Tabasco (or similar chili sauce)
- 2 tbsp. pumpkin seeds (or roasted sunflower seeds, to use as garnish)
- ½ bunch mint, fresh

Directions:

1. Using vegetable broth for the tastiest results, cook the couscous according to packet instructions. Now add hot vegetable broth to it until it is all filled with the couscous.
2. Position a tea-towel over the end. Give it a slight swirl after 3-4 minutes to make it fluffy. For 1 more minute, cover again.
3. Rub the carrots and dice the cucumber, peppers, tomatoes (fresh and sun-dried), mint, and parsley in the meantime.
4. With the cooked couscous, add the lemon juice, tomato paste, olive oil, salt, pepper, Tabasco sauce, and chopped and grated vegetables and herbs. Mix and serve. If using, garnish with seeds.

Nutrition:

Calories: 80 Carbs: 6g

Fat: 5g Protein: 1g

142. Easy Cauliflower Curry

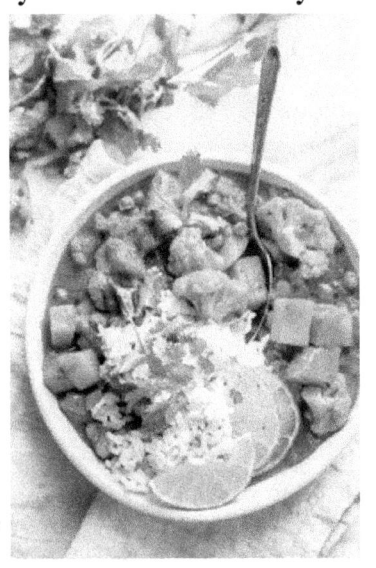

Preparation time: 10 minutes

Cooking time: 20 minutes

Servings: 4

Level of difficulty: Normal

Category: Green

Ingredients:

- 1 bunch cilantro/coriander, fresh
- 1 tbsp. maple syrup
- 1 tbsp. curry powder
- 1 lime (juiced)
- 1 can of coconut milk
- ½ tbsp. curry paste
- 1 tbsp. olive oil
- 2 thumbs ginger, fresh
- 1 cup green beans

- 1 small-medium potato
- ½ red peppers
- onions
- Salt
- ½ medium cauliflowers

Directions:

1. Cut the cauliflower into bite-sized bits; slice the potatoes and bell pepper into small pieces. The tips of the green beans are separated and sliced in two.

2. Dice the onion and slice the ginger finely. Add some oil to a pan and add the ginger over medium heat.

3. Add the onion and bell pepper as soon as it begins to release its scent (about 2 minutes) and sauté (fry over medium heat) for 5 minutes. Mix in the paste of the curry, stir and simmer for another 2 minutes.

4. To dissolve the curry paste, stir in a little coconut milk and then add the remainder. Set to high heat before the milk begins to boil.

5. Reduce to low heat and apply lime juice, curry powder, salt, and maple syrup until boiling. Only mix well.

6. Now it is time for the potatoes and cauliflower to be added. Simmer for 5 minutes, add the green beans and leave to simmer for another 5 minutes.

7. Give a taste test to the curry: see if you need any more salt, sugar, or lime to apply. You can even add a little more curry paste as well. It's ready to serve until you're comfortable.

8. Serve on top of sliced new cilantro. With this lovely curry meal, rice or quinoa goes well!

Nutrition:

Calories: 475

Carbs: 45g

Fat: 24g

Protein: 26g

CHAPTER 10:

Soups and Salads

143. Swiss Cheese and Broccoli Soup

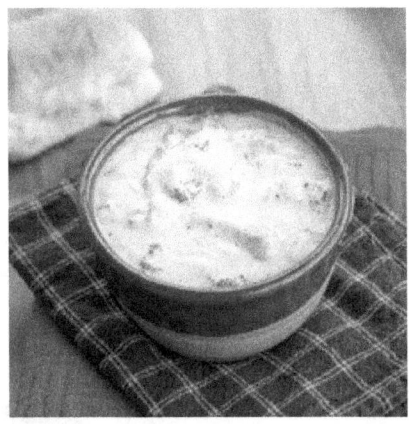

Preparation time: 5 minutes

Cooking time: 15 minutes

Servings: 8

Level of difficulty: Normal

Category: Green

Ingredients:

- 4 cups water, divided
- 4 teaspoons chicken bouillon granules
- 6 cups frozen chopped broccoli
- 4 cups of milk
- 1/2 teaspoon salt
- 1/4 teaspoon pepper
- 1/8 teaspoon ground nutmeg
- 1/2 cup all-purpose flour
- 1-1/4 cups shredded Swiss cheese
- 3/4 cup shredded cheddar cheese

Directions:

1. In a 4- to 5-quart skillet, cook broccoli in 2 cups boiling water for about 5 minutes or until tender. Drain; set aside.
2. To the same skillet, add milk, salt, pepper, nutmeg, and remaining water. Stir in flour; cook and stir until thickened and bubbly. Stir in broccoli; heat through.
3. Preheat oven to 450F. Add Swiss and cheddar cheeses, stirring until melted. Pour into a 2-quart casserole.
4. Bake for 5 to 8 minutes or until cheese is melted. Ladle hot soup into bowls; garnish with desired toppings and serve.

Nutrition:

Calories: 273 Protein: 18.1 g

Fat: 12.21 g

Carbohydrates: 24.62 g

144. Tavern Soup

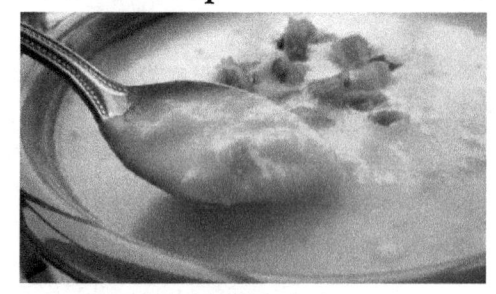

Preparation time: 15 minutes

Cooking time: 3 hours

Servings: 6

Level of difficulty: Normal

Category: Green

Ingredients:

- 1 stalk celery thinly sliced
- 1 carrot peeled and sliced thin
- 1/4 cup finely chopped green pepper(optional)
- 1 small onion finely chopped
- 42 oz chicken broth
- 12 oz of beer at room temp
- 1/2 tsp salt
- 1/4 tsp pepper
- 5 tbsp cornstarch
- 1/4 cup water
- 1 cup sharp cheddar cheese shredded

Directions:

1. Put the vegetables in the bottom of your pot. Add chicken broth and beer. Cook on high for 1 hour. Add the rest of the ingredients except cheese.
2. Cook on high an additional 2 hours. Shred cheddar cheese. Turn pot to low, add cheese and stir until cheese looks like melted butter. Then serve with crackers.

Nutrition:

Calories: 388

Protein: 37.59 g

Fat: 19.74 g

Carbohydrates: 11.28 g

145. Broccoli Blue Cheese

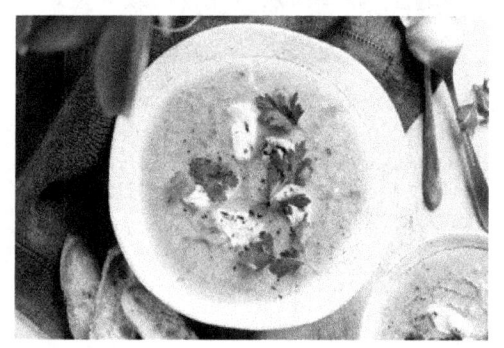

Preparation time: 15 minutes

Cooking time: 15 minutes

Servings: 4

Level of difficulty: Normal

Category: Green

Ingredients:

- 3 tablespoons unsalted butter
- 1 small onion, chopped

- 1 1/2 pounds broccoli florets
- 2 cups reduced-sodium chicken broth
- 1/2 cup crumbled gorgonzola cheese, divided
- 1/2 teaspoon salt
- 1/2 teaspoon pepper
- 3/4 cup half-and-half
- 1/2 cup croutons

Directions:

1. In a large stockpot, heat butter over medium-high heat; cook onion, stirring, until softened, about 5 minutes. Add broth, broccoli, 1/2 cup cheese, 1/2 teaspoon salt, and 1/2 teaspoon pepper to the pot.
2. Cover, adjust the heat to medium-low, then simmer until broccoli is just tender, about 5 minutes. Remove pot from heat; let broccoli stand for 4 minutes.
3. Stir in half-and-half; cook over medium heat until heated through, about 1 minute. Stir in croutons; divide among soup bowls. Sprinkle with remaining 1/4 cup cheese.

Nutrition:

Calories: 391

Protein: 37.59 g

Fat: 20.8 g

Carbohydrates: 14.72 g

146. Cream of Mushroom Soup

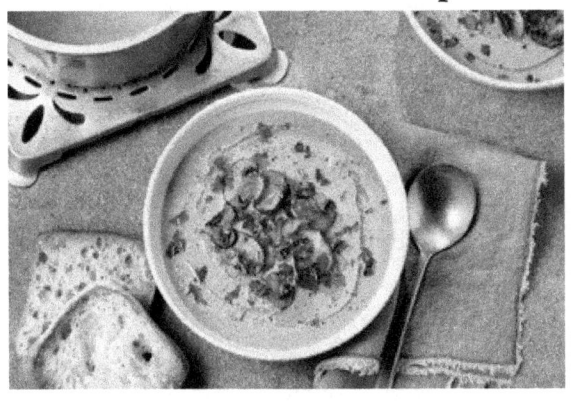

Preparation time: 10 minutes

Cooking time: 30 minutes

Servings: 6

Level of difficulty: Normal

Category: Green

Ingredients:

- 4 tablespoons butter
- 1 tablespoon oil
- 2 onions diced
- 4 cloves garlic minced
- 1 1/2 pounds (750 g) fresh brown mushrooms sliced
- 4 teaspoons chopped thyme divided
- 1/2 cup Marsala wine (any dry red or white wine)
- 6 tablespoons all-purpose flour
- 4 cups low-sodium chicken broth or stock
- 1-2 teaspoons salt adjust to taste

- 1/2-1 teaspoons black cracked pepper adjust to taste
- 2 beef bouillon cubes, crumbled
- 1 cup heavy cream or half and a half (sub with evaporated milk)
- Chopped fresh parsley and thyme to serve

Directions:

1. Warm oven to 375 degrees Fahrenheit (190 degrees Celsius).
2. Sweat diced onions and minced garlic in butter and oil in a thick-bottomed saucepan for about 5 minutes, until onions are translucent. Add in sliced mushrooms, 2 teaspoons of chopped thyme, and Marsala wine.
3. Toss to combine, then cook until mushrooms are tender. Add in flour and cook for another few minutes and then gradually add in chicken broth. Stir in heavy cream and bring to a gentle boil. Stir occasionally.
4. Drop crumbled bouillon cubes. Add the leftover thyme, 1 teaspoon salt, and pepper to taste. Cook for 25-30 minutes until thickened. Adjust seasonings and serve with fresh chopped parsley and thyme.

Nutrition:

Calories: 227

Protein: 11.24 g

Fat: 12.78 g

Carbohydrates: 20.16 g

147. Olive Soup

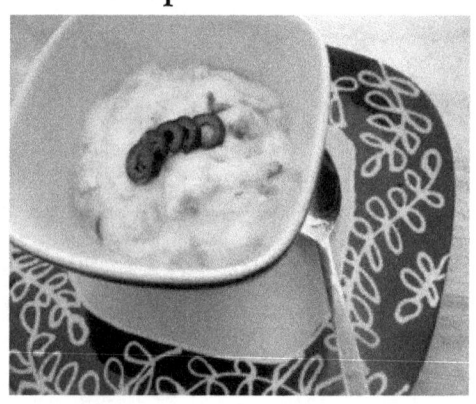

Preparation time: 30 minutes

Cooking time: 40 minutes

Servings: 8

Level of difficulty: Normal

Category: Green

Ingredients:

- 4 tablespoons butter
- 1/4 cup sweet onion diced
- 1/4 cup carrot diced
- 1/4 cup celery diced
- 2 tablespoons flour
- 4 cups chicken stock
- 1 cup white wine
- 1 1/2 cups half and half
- 1/2 cup cooked white rice
- 1/4 cup each sliced large black and pimento-stuffed green olives
- 1/4 cup frozen peas

- 2 cups chicken breast, cooked, cut into bite-sized pieces
- White pepper and salt if needed

Directions:

1. Melt the butter in a 3 or 5-quart saucepan over medium-low heat. Add the onions, carrot, and celery, and cook for about 10 minutes until tender.
2. Start stirring in the flour and cook for about 5 minutes. Slowly stir in the chicken stock and white wine and bring to a boil.
3. In a medium bowl, whisk the half and half until it has at least doubled in volume. Add this to the soup.
4. Cook for about 15 minutes, occasionally whisking until thickened. Stir in the rice, black olives, green olives, peas, chicken, and any other vegetables you want to add.
5. Add pepper and salt to taste. Allow to chill in the refrigerator within 4 hours or preferably overnight. Reheat the soup if needed. Garnish with a sprinkling of minced fresh parsley. Enjoy!

Nutrition:

Calories: 669

Protein: 100.41 g

Fat: 21.08 g

Carbohydrates: 13.51 g

148. Normandy Salad

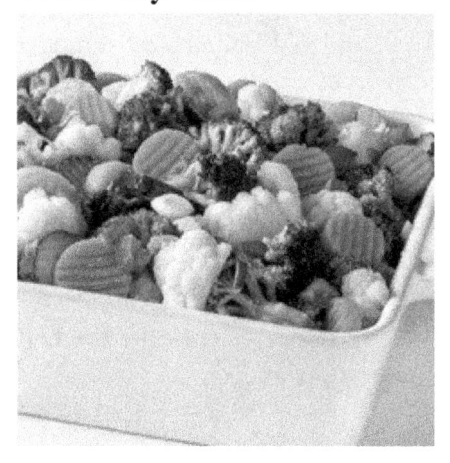

Preparation Time: 25 minutes

Cooking Time: 5 minutes

Servings: 4 to 6

Level of difficulty: Normal

Category: Green

Ingredients:

For the walnuts:

- 2 tablespoons butter
- ¼ cup sugar or honey
- 1 cup walnut pieces
- ½ teaspoon kosher salt

For the dressing:

- 3 tablespoons extra-virgin olive oil
- 1½ tablespoons champagne vinegar
- 1½ tablespoons Dijon mustard
- ¼ teaspoon kosher salt

For the salad:

- 1 head red leaf lettuce, shredded into pieces
- 3 heads endive, ends trimmed and leaves separated
- 2 apples, cored and divided into thin wedges
- 1 (8-ounce) Camembert wheel, cut into thin wedges

Directions:

1. For the walnuts, dissolve the butter in a skillet over medium-high heat. Stir in the sugar and cook until it dissolves.
2. Add the walnuts and cook for about 5 minutes, stirring, until toasty. Season with salt and transfer to a plate to cool.
3. For the dressing, whip the oil, vinegar, mustard, and salt in a large bowl until combined.
4. For the salad, add the lettuce and endive to the bowl with the dressing, and toss to coat. Transfer to a serving platter.
5. Decoratively arrange the apple and Camembert wedges over the lettuce and scatter the walnuts on top. Serve immediately.

Nutrition:

Calories: 699 Fat: 52 g

Carbs: 44 g

Protein: 23 g

149. Loaded Caesar Salad with Crunchy Chickpeas

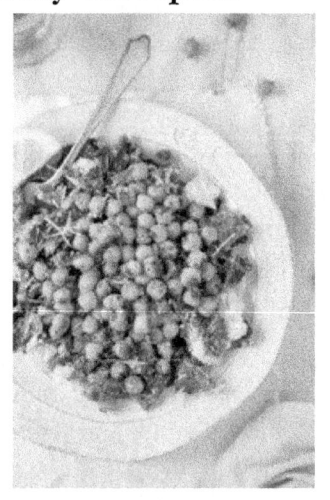

Preparation Time: 5 minutes

Cooking Time: 20 minutes

Servings: 6

Level of difficulty: Normal

Category: Green

Ingredients:

For the chickpeas:

- 2 (15-ounce) cans chickpeas, drained and rinsed
- 2 tablespoons extra-virgin olive oil
- 1 teaspoon kosher salt
- 1 teaspoon garlic powder
- 1 teaspoon onion powder
- 1 teaspoon dried oregano

For the dressing:

- ½ cup mayonnaise

- 2 tablespoons grated Parmesan cheese
- 2 tablespoons freshly squeezed lemon juice
- 1 clove garlic, peeled and smashed
- 1 teaspoon Dijon mustard
- ½ tablespoon Worcestershire sauce
- ½ tablespoon anchovy paste

For the salad:

- 3 heads romaine lettuce, cut into bite-size pieces

Directions:

1. For the chickpeas, warm the oven to 450°F. Line a baking sheet with parchment paper.
2. Add the chickpeas, oil, salt, garlic powder, onion powder, and oregano in a small container. Scatter the coated chickpeas on the prepared baking sheet.
3. Roast for about 20 minutes, occasionally tossing, until the chickpeas are golden and have a bit of crunch.
4. For the dressing, whisk the mayonnaise, Parmesan, lemon juice, garlic, mustard, Worcestershire sauce, and anchovy paste until combined in a small bowl.
5. For the salad, combine the lettuce and dressing in a large container. Toss to coat. Top with the roasted chickpeas and serve.

Nutrition:

Calories: 367

Fat: 22 g

Carbs: 35 g

Protein: 12 g

150. Coleslaw Worth A Second Helping

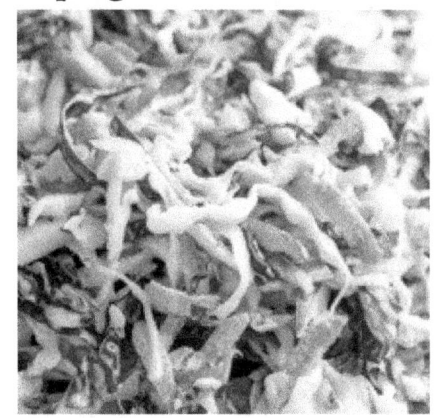

Preparation Time: 20 minutes

Cooking Time: 10 minutes

Servings: 6

Level of difficulty: Easy

Category: Green

Ingredients:

- 5 cups shredded cabbage
- 2 carrots, shredded
- ½ cup mayonnaise
- ½ cup sour cream
- 3 tablespoons apple cider vinegar

- 1 teaspoon kosher salt
- ½ teaspoon celery seed

Directions:
1. Add together the cabbage, carrots, and parsley in a large bowl. Whisk together the mayonnaise, sour cream, vinegar, salt, and celery in a small bowl until smooth.
2. Pour sauce over veggies until covered. Transfer to a serving bowl and bake until ready to serve.

Nutrition:

Calories: 192

Fat: 18 g

Carbs: 7 g

Protein: 2 g

151. Romaine Lettuce and Radicchios Mix

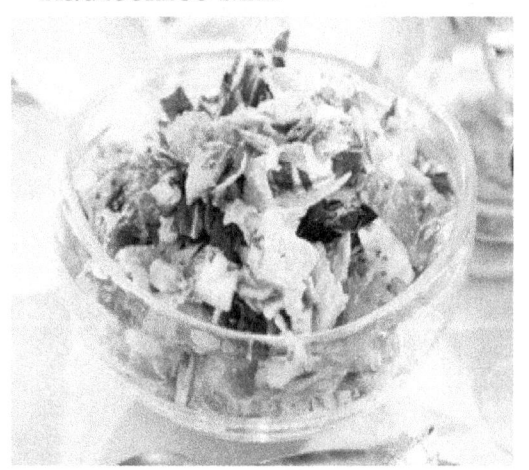

Preparation Time: 6 minutes

Cooking Time: 0 minutes

Servings: 4

Level of difficulty: Easy

Category: Green

Ingredients:
- 2 tablespoons olive oil
- A pinch of salt and black pepper
- 2 spring onions, chopped
- 3 tablespoons Dijon mustard
- Juice of 1 lime
- ½ cup basil, chopped
- 4 cups romaine lettuce heads, chopped
- 3 radicchios, sliced

Directions:
1. In a salad bowl, blend the lettuce with the spring onions and the other ingredients. Toss and serve.

Nutrition:

Calories: 87

Fats: 2 g

Carbs: 1 g

Protein: 2 g

152. Greek Salad

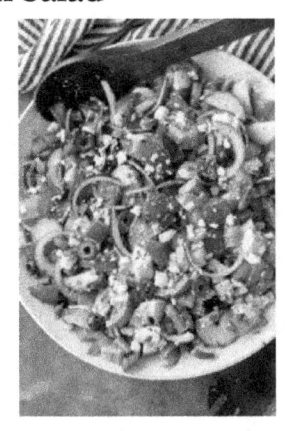

Preparation Time: 15 minutes

Cooking Time: 0 minutes

Servings: 5

Level of difficulty: Easy

Category: Green

Ingredients:

For Dressing: ½ teaspoon black pepper

- ¼ teaspoon salt
- ½ teaspoon oregano
- 1 tablespoon garlic powder
- 2 tablespoons balsamic vinegar
- 1/3 cup olive oil

For Salad: ½ cup sliced black olives

- ½ cup chopped parsley, fresh
- 1 small red onion, thin-sliced
- 1 cup cherry tomatoes, sliced
- 1 bell pepper, yellow, chunked
- 1 cucumber, peeled, quarter and slice
- 4 cups chopped romaine lettuce
- ½ teaspoon salt
- 2 tablespoons olive oil

Directions:

1. In a small container, mix all fixings for the dressing and let this set in the freezer while you make the salad.
2. To assemble the salad, mix all the ingredients in a large-sized bowl and toss the veggies gently but thoroughly to combine. Serve the salad with the dressing as you desire.

Nutrition: Calories: 234 Fat: 16.1 g Protein: 5 g Carbs: 48 g

153. Asparagus and Smoked Salmon Salad

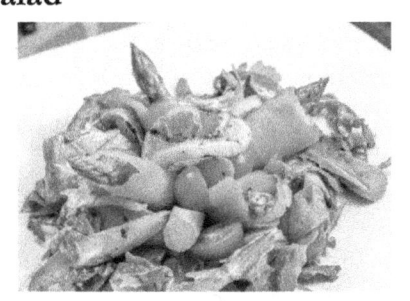

Preparation Time: 15 minutes

Cooking Time: 10 minutes

Servings: 8

Level of difficulty: Normal

Category: Lean

Ingredients:

- 1 lb. fresh asparagus, shaped and cut into 1-inch pieces

- 1/2 cup pecans, smashed into pieces
- 2 heads red leaf lettuce, washed and split
- 1/2 cup frozen green peas, thawed
- 1/4 lb. smoked salmon, cut into 1-inch chunks
- 1/4 cup olive oil
- 2 tablespoons lemon juice
- 1 teaspoon Dijon mustard
- 1/2 teaspoon salt
- 1/4 teaspoon pepper

Directions:
1. Boil a pot of water. Stir in asparagus and cook for 5 minutes until tender. Let it drain and set aside.
2. In a skillet, cook the pecans over medium heat for 5 minutes, continually stirring until lightly toasted.
3. Combine the asparagus, toasted pecans, salmon, peas, and red leaf lettuce and toss in a large bowl.
4. In another bowl, combine lemon juice, pepper, Dijon mustard, salt, and olive oil. You can coat the salad with the dressing, then serve.

Nutrition:

Calories: 159 Carbs: 7 g

Fat: 12.9 g

Protein: 6 g

154. Shrimp Cobb Salad

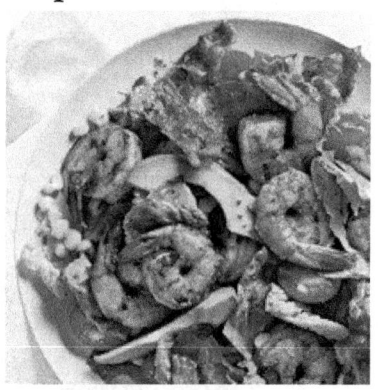

Preparation Time: 25 minutes

Cooking Time: 10 minutes

Servings: 2

Level of difficulty: Normal

Category: Leanest

Ingredients:

- 4 slices center-cut bacon
- 1 lb. large shrimp, peeled and deveined
- 1/2 teaspoon ground paprika
- 1/4 teaspoon ground black pepper
- 1/4 teaspoon salt, divided
- 2 1/2 tablespoons fresh lemon juice
- 1 1/2 tablespoons extra-virgin olive oil
- 1/2 teaspoon whole-grain Dijon mustard
- 1 (10 oz.) package romaine lettuce hearts, chopped
- 2 cups cherry tomatoes, quartered

- 1 ripe avocado, cut into wedges
- 1 cup shredded carrots

Directions:

1. Cook the bacon for 4 minutes on each side in a large skillet over medium heat till crispy.
2. Take away from the skillet and place on paper towels; let cool for 5 minutes. Break the bacon into bits. Throw out most of the bacon fat, leaving behind only 1 tablespoon in the skillet.
3. Bring the skillet back to medium-high heat. Add black pepper and paprika to the shrimp for seasoning.
4. Cook the shrimp for around 2 minutes on each side until it is opaque. Sprinkle with 1/8 teaspoon of salt for seasoning.
5. Combine the remaining 1/8 teaspoon of salt, mustard, olive oil, and lemon juice in a small bowl. Stir in the romaine hearts.
6. On each serving plate, place 1 and 1/2 cups of romaine lettuce. Add on top the same amounts of avocado, carrots, tomatoes, shrimp, and bacon.

Nutrition:

Calories: 528

Carbohydrate: 22.7 g

Fat: 28.7 g

Protein: 48.9 g

LEAN AND GREEN DIET COOKBOOK:

CHAPTER 11:

Snacks

155. Bacon Cheeseburger

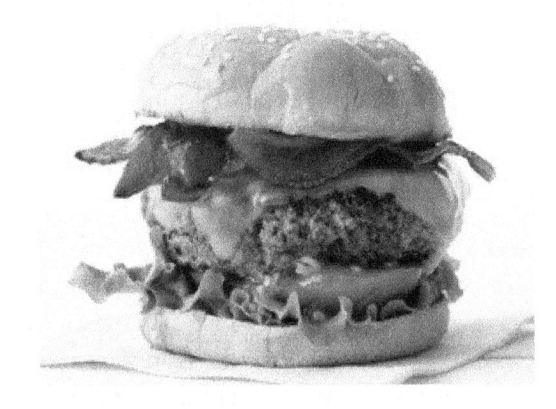

Preparation Time: 10 Minutes

Cooking Time: 30 Minutes

Servings: 4

Level of difficulty: Normal

Category: Lean

Ingredients:

- 1 lb. lean ground beef
- 1/4 cup chopped yellow onion
- 1 garlic clove, minced
- 1 tbsp. yellow mustard
- 1 tbsp. Worcestershire sauce
- 1/2 tsp. salt
- cooking spray
- 4 ultra-thin slices of cheddar cheese, cut into six equal-sized rectangular pieces
- 3 pieces of turkey bacon, each cut into eight evenly-sized rectangular pieces
- 24 dill pickle chips
- 4-6 green leaf
- lettuce leaves, torn into 24 small square-shaped pieces
- 12 cherry tomatoes, sliced in half

Directions:

1. Pre-heat oven to 400°F. Combine the garlic, salt, onion, Worcestershire sauce, and beef in a medium-sized bowl, and mix well.
2. Form mixture into 24 small meatballs. Put meatballs onto a foil-lined baking sheet and cook for 12-15 minutes. Leave oven on.
3. Top every meatball with a piece of cheese, then go back to the oven until cheese melts for about 2 to 3 minutes. Let meatballs cool.

4. To assemble the bites: on a toothpick layer, a cheese-covered meatball, piece of bacon, piece of lettuce, pickle chip, and a tomato half.

Nutrition:

Calories: 500

Carbs: 29g

Fat: 30g

Protein: 27g

156. Cheeseburger Pie

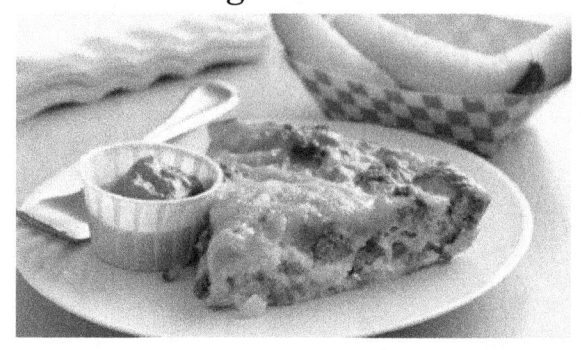

Preparation Time: 20 Minutes

Cooking Time: 90 Minutes

Servings: 4

Level of difficulty: Normal

Category: Lean

Ingredients:

- 1 large spaghetti squash
- 1 lb. lean ground beef
- 1/4 cup diced onion
- 2 eggs
- 1/3 cup low-fat, plain Greek yogurt
- 2 tbsp. tomato sauce
- 1/2 tsp. Worcestershire sauce
- 2/3 cup reduced-fat, shredded cheddar cheese
- 2 oz. dill pickle slices
- Cooking spray

Directions:

1. Preheat oven to 400°F. Slice spaghetti squash in half lengthwise; dismiss pulp and seeds. Spray insides with cooking spray.

2. Place squash halves cut-side-down onto a foil-lined baking sheet, and bake for 30 minutes. Once cooked, let cool before scraping squash flesh with a fork to remove spaghetti-like strands; set aside.

3. Push squash strands in the bottom and up sides of the greased pie pan, creating an even layer.

4. Meanwhile, set up pie filling. In a lightly greased, medium-sized skillet, cook beef and onion over medium heat for 8 to 10 minutes, sometimes stirring, until meat is brown. Drain and remove from heat.

5. In a medium-sized bowl, whisk together eggs, tomato paste, Greek yogurt, and Worcestershire sauce. Stir in ground beef mixture.

6. Pour pie filling over squash crust. Sprinkle meat filling with cheese, and

then top with dill pickle slices—Bake for 40 minutes. Serve.

Nutrition:

Calories: 409

Fat: 24.49g

Carbohydrates: 15.06g

Protein: 30.69g

157. Personal Pizza Biscuit

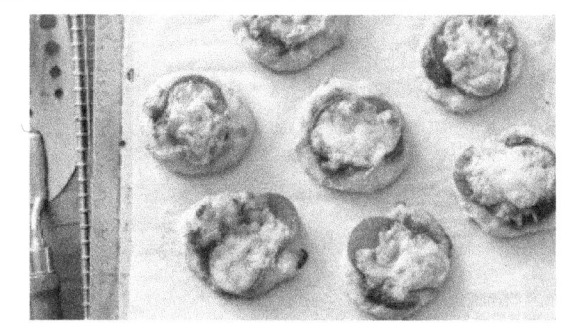

Preparation Time: 5 Minutes

Cooking Time: 15 Minutes

Servings: 1

Level of difficulty: Easy

Category: Green

Ingredients:

- 1 sachet Lean and Green select
- buttermilk cheddar herb biscuit
- 2 tbsp cold water
- cooking spray
- 2 tbsp no-sugar-added tomato sauce
- 1/4 cup reduced-fat shredded cheese

Directions:

1. Preheat oven to 350°F. Mix biscuit and water, and spread mixture into a small, circular crust shape onto a greased, foil-lined baking sheet.
2. Bake for 10 minutes. Top with tomato sauce and cheese, and cook till cheese is melted, about 5 minutes.

Nutrition:

Calories: 500 Carbs: 31g

Fat: 25g Protein: 11g

158. Chicken and Mushrooms

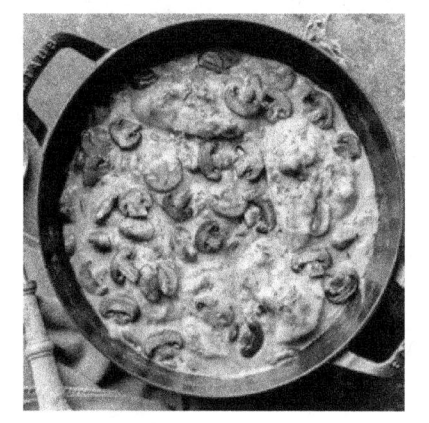

Preparation Time: 10 Minutes

Cooking Time: 15 Minutes

Servings: 6

Level of difficulty: Normal

Category: Leaner

Ingredients:

- 2 breasts of chicken
- 1 cup of sliced white champignons

- 1 cup of sliced green chilies
- 1/2 cup scallions hacked
- 1 teaspoon of chopped garlic
- 1 cup of low-fat cheddar shredded cheese (1-1,5 lb. grams fat / ounce)
- 1 tablespoon of olive oil
- 1 tablespoon of butter

Directions:

1. Fry the chicken breasts with olive oil. When needed, add salt and pepper. Grill breasts of chicken on a plate with grill.
2. Weigh 4 ounces of chicken for every serving. (Makes two servings, save leftovers for another meal).
3. In a buttered pan, stir in mushrooms, green peppers, scallions, and garlic until smooth and a little dark. Place the chicken on a baking platter.
4. Cover with the mushroom combination—top on ham. Place the cheese in a 350C oven until it melts.

Nutrition:

Calories: 258

Carbs: 13g

Fat: 12g

Protein: 0g

159. Chicken Enchilada Bake

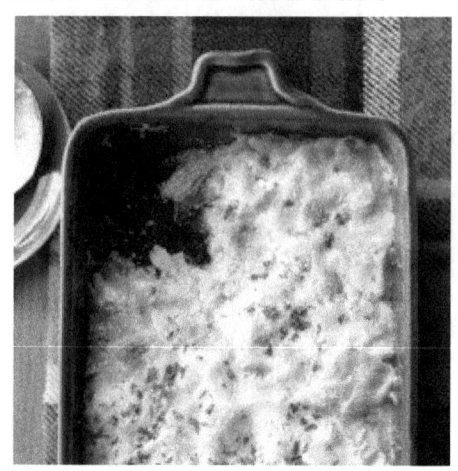

Preparation Time: 20 Minutes

Cooking Time: 50 Minutes

Servings: 5

Level of difficulty: Normal

Category: Leaner

Ingredients:

- 5 oz. shredded chicken breast or 99 percent fat-free white chicken can be used in a pan
- 1 can tomatoes paste
- 1 low sodium chicken broth can be fat-free
- 1/4 cup-cheese with low-fat mozzarella
- 1 tablespoon -oil
- 1 tbsp of salt
- ground cumin, chili powder, garlic powder, oregano, and onion powder (all to taste).

- 1 to 2 zucchinis sliced longways
- Sliced olives (optional)

Directions:

1. Prepare Enchilada Sauce: add olive oil in a saucepan over medium/high heat, stir in tomato paste and seasonings, and heat in chicken broth for 2-3 minutes.
2. Stirring regularly to boil, turn heat to low for 15 minutes. Set aside & cool to ambient temperature.
3. Pull-strip of Zucchini through enchilada sauce and lay flat on the pan's bottom in a small baking pan, spray with Pam.
4. Add the chicken a little less than 1/4 cup of enchilada sauce and mix it. Stick the chicken to the lids, side to side of the baking dish.
5. Sprinkle over chicken with some bacon. Add another layer of the pulled zucchini via enchilada sauce (similar to lasagna making).
6. When needed, cover with the remaining cheese and olives on top. Bake it for 35 to 40 minutes. Keep an eye on them. When the cheese begins burning, cover with foil.

Nutrition:

Calories: 312

Carbohydrates: 21.3g

Protein: 27g

Fat: 10.2g

160. Jalapeno Lentil (Chickpea) Burgers + Avocado Mango Pico

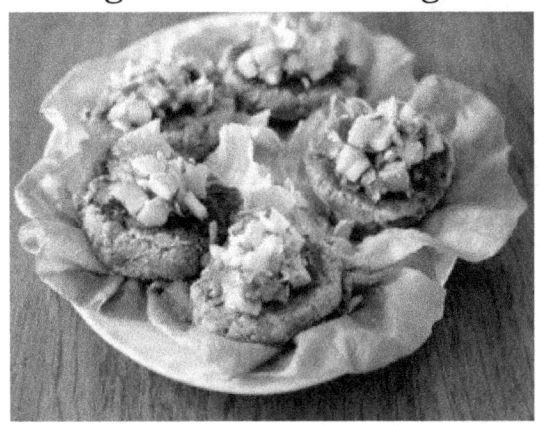

Preparation Time: 15 Minutes

Cooking Time: 10 Minutes

Servings: 5

Level of difficulty: Normal

Category: Green

Ingredients:

- ½ cup dried red lentils, rinsed
- 1 can chickpeas; rinsed
- 1 tsp ground cumin
- 1 tsp chili powder
- 1 tsp sea salt
- ½ cup packed cilantro
- garlic cloves minced
- jalapeno finely chopped
- ½ red onion, small, minced
- red bell pepper
- carrot, shredded

- ¼ cup oat bran/oat flour (gluten-free)
- lettuce/hamburger buns

For Pico:

- 1 ripe mango, diced
- 1 ripe avocado, diced
- ½ red onion, small, finely diced
- ½ cup chopped cilantro
- ½ tsp fresh lime juice
- sea salt

Directions:

1. Put all fixings in a large bowl and mix. Stir in the salt to taste. Put a medium saucepan on medium heat, add lentils plus 1 1/2 cups of water, then bring water to a boil, cover it afterward, lower the heat to low, and then simmer lentils until the water is absorbed. Drain, and set aside some extra water.
2. In a food processor, put the cooked lentils, chickpeas, garlic, sea salt, cilantro, chili powder, and cumin, and blend until the beans and lentils are smooth.
3. Add tomato, red pepper, jalapeno, and carrot to compare. Divide into six equal parts and use your hands to create dense patties.
4. Heat skillet over a medium-high flame; apply 1/2 tablespoon of olive oil. Place a few burgers in at a time and cook on either side for a couple of minutes, just until crisp and golden brown.
5. Repeat with remaining patties and add olive oil whenever desired. Place the patties in a bun or lettuce and finish with mango avocado Pico.

Nutrition:

Calories: 225

Carbs: 35g

Fat: 6g

Protein: 10g

161. Grandma's Rice

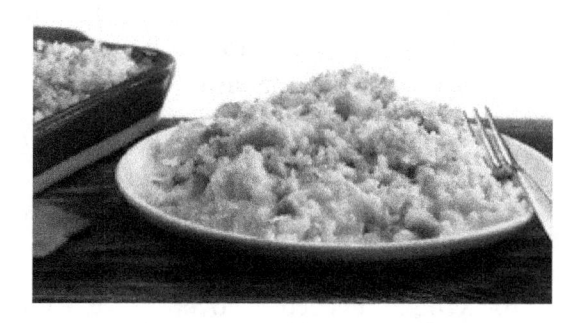

Preparation time: 15 minutes

Cooking time: 2 hours

Servings: 4

Level of difficulty: Normal

Category: Green

Ingredients:

- 40g butter
- 1/2 cup brown sugar

- 1/2 cup arborio rice
- 3 cups of milk
- 1/2 tbsp ground cinnamon
- 1/8 tbsp ground nutmeg
- 1 tbsp vanilla paste
- 1/2 cup raisins
- 300ml cream

Directions:

1. Preheat oven to 300F. Grease a 1-liter ability oven-proof dish. Heat butter in a saucepan and add sugar and rice.
2. Stir for 1 minute to thoroughly coat the rice. Remove from heat and wish in milk, spices, and vanilla. Stir through raisins, then pour into the prepared dish.
3. Bake for 30 minutes, then remove from the oven and stir well. Drizzle over the cream and return to the oven for an additional hour.
4. Check that rice is cooked through. Return to the oven for 15-30 minutes if required. Serve with extra cream and nutmeg.

Nutrition:

Calories: 197

Fat: 20g

Protein: 23g

Carbohydrates: 30g

162. Baked Beef Zucchini

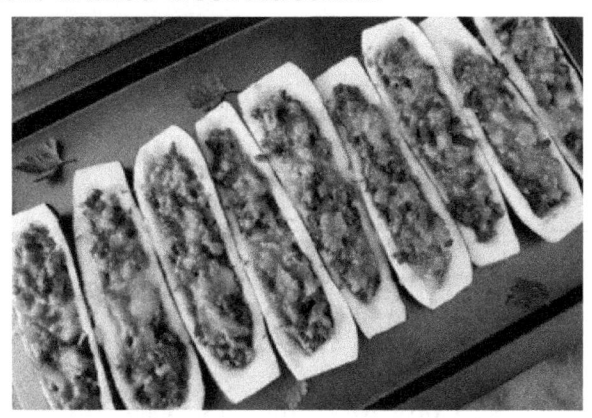

Preparation Time: 10 minutes

Cooking Time: 40 minutes

Servings: 4

Level of difficulty: Normal

Category: Lean

Ingredients:

- 2 large zucchinis
- 1 cup minced beef
- 1 cup mushroom, chopped
- 1 tomato, chopped
- 1/2 cup spinach, chopped
- 1 tbsp chives, minced
- 2 tbsp olive oil
- salt and pepper to taste
- 1 tbsp almond butter
- 1 tsp. garlic powder
- 1 cup cheddar cheese, grated
- 1/3 tsp. ginger powder

Directions:

1. Warm oven to 400 degrees F. Add aluminum foil on a baking sheet. Cut the zucchini in half. Scoop out the seeds and make pockets to stuff it later.
2. In a pan, add the olive oil. Toss the beef until brown. Add the mushroom, tomato, chives, salt, pepper, garlic, ginger, and spinach.
3. Cook for 2 minutes. Take off the heat. Stuff the zucchinis using the mix. Add them onto the baking sheet, then sprinkle the cheese on top. Add the butter on top, bake for 30 minutes. Serve warm.

Nutrition:

Calories: 100 Fat: 12.8g

Carbohydrate: 26.8g Protein: 0g

163. Baked Tuna with Asparagus

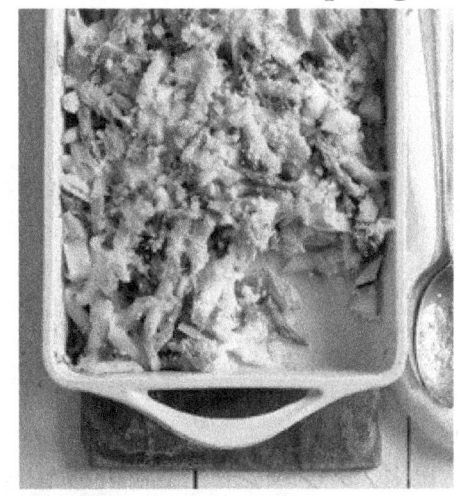

Preparation time: 10 minutes

Cooking time: 10 minutes

Servings: 2

Level of difficulty: Normal

Category: Leanest

Ingredients:

- 2 tuna steaks
- 1 cup asparagus, trimmed
- 1 tsp. almond butter
- 1 tsp. rosemary
- 1/2 tsp. oregano
- 1/2 tsp. garlic powder
- 1 tsp. lemon juice
- 1/2 tsp. ginger powder
- 1 tbsp. olive oil
- 1 tsp. red chili powder
- salt and pepper to taste

Directions:

1. Marinate the tuna using oregano, lemon juice, salt, pepper, red chili powder, garlic, ginger, and let it sit for 10 minutes.
2. In a pan, add the olive oil. Fry the tuna steaks within 2 minutes per side. In another pan, melt the almond butter. Toss the asparagus with salt, pepper, and rosemary for 3 minutes. Serve.

Nutrition:

Calories: 153 Fat: 4.7g

Protein: 27g Carbohydrate: 3.2g

164. Lamb Stuffed Avocado

Preparation Time: 10 Minutes

Cooking Time: 40 Minutes

Servings: 4

Level of difficulty: Normal

Category: Lean

Ingredients:

- 2 avocados
- 1 1/2 cup minced lamb
- 1/2 cup cheddar cheese, grated
- 1/2 cup parmesan cheese, grated
- 2 tbsp. almond, chopped
- 1 tbsp. coriander, chopped
- 2 tbsp. olive oil
- 1 tomato, chopped
- 1 jalapeno, chopped
- salt and pepper to taste
- 1 tsp. garlic, chopped
- 1 -inch ginger piece, chopped

Directions:

1. Cut the avocados in half. Remove the pit and scoop out some flesh to stuff it later. In a skillet, add half of the oil. Toss the ginger, garlic for 1 minute.
2. Add the lamb and toss for 3 minutes. Add the tomato, coriander, parmesan, jalapeno, salt, pepper, and cook for 2 minutes.
3. Take off the heat. Stuff the avocados. Sprinkle the almonds, cheddar cheese, and add olive oil on top. Add to a baking sheet and bake for 30 minutes. Serve.

Nutrition:

Calories: 298 Fat: 19.5g

Protein: 21g Carbohydrate: 13.1g

165. Sweet Almond Bites

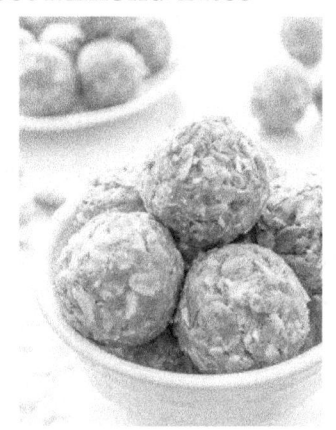

Preparation Time: 30 minutes

Cooking Time: 2 minutes

Servings: 12

Level of difficulty: Easy

Category: Healthy Fat

Ingredients:

- 18 ounces butter, grass-fed
- 2 ounces heavy cream
- ½ cup stevia
- 2/3 cup cocoa powder
- 1 teaspoon vanilla extract, pure

- 4 tablespoons almond butter

Directions:

1. Use a double boiler to dissolve your butter before adding in all of your remaining ingredients. Place the mixture into molds, freezing for two hours before serving.

Nutrition: Calories: 350 Protein: 2

Fat: 38 Carbs: 42g

166. Strawberry Cheesecake Minis

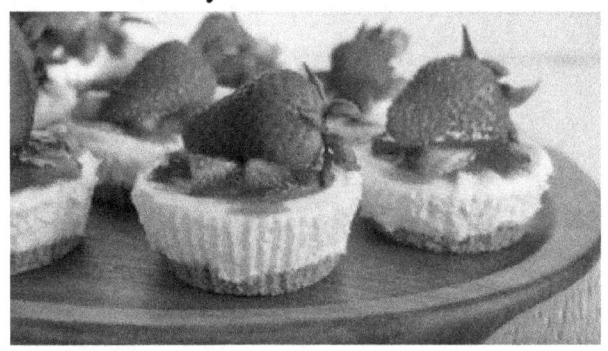

Preparation Time: 30 minutes

Cooking Time: 0 minutes

Servings: 12

Level of difficulty: Easy

Category: Healthy Fat

Ingredients:

- 1 cup of coconut oil
- 1 cup coconut butter
- ½ cup strawberries, sliced
- ½ teaspoon lime juice
- 2 tablespoons cream cheese, full fat
- stevia to taste

Directions:

1. Blend your strawberries. Soften your cream cheese, and then add in your coconut butter. Combine all ingredients, and then pour your mixture into silicone molds. Freeze for at least two hours before serving.

Nutrition: Calories: 372 Protein: 1 g

Fat: 41 g Carbohydrates: 2 g

167. Cocoa Brownies

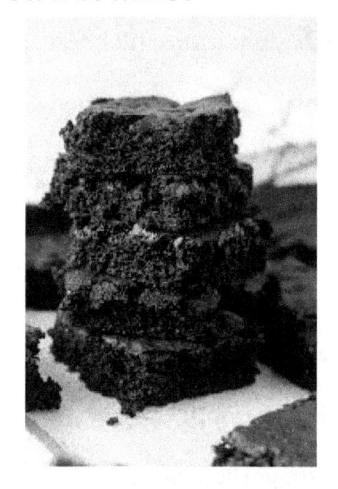

Preparation Time: 10 minutes

Cooking Time: 30 minutes

Level of difficulty: Normal

Servings: 12

Category: Healthy Fat

Ingredients:

- 1 egg
- 2 tablespoons butter, grass-fed

- 2 teaspoons vanilla extract, pure
- ¼ teaspoon baking powder
- ¼ cup of cocoa powder
- 1/3 cup heavy cream
- ¾ cup almond butter
- pinch sea salt

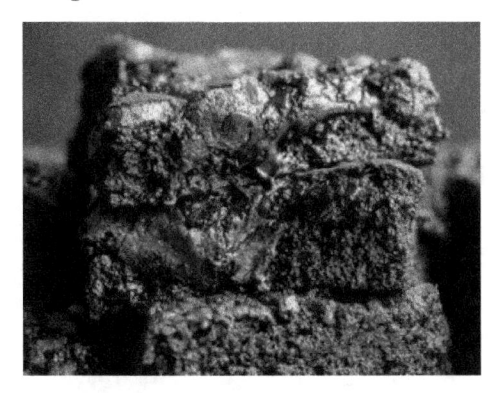

Directions:

1. Break your egg into a bowl, whisking until smooth. Add in all of your wet ingredients, mixing well. Mix all dry ingredients into a bowl.
2. Sift your dry ingredients into your wet ingredients, mixing to form a batter. Get out a baking pan, greasing it before pouring in your mixture.
3. Warm your oven to 350 F and bake within 25 minutes. Allow it to cool before slicing and serve room temperature or warm.

Nutrition:

Calories: 184 Protein: 1g

Fat: 20g

Carbohydrates: 1g

168. Chocolate Orange Bites

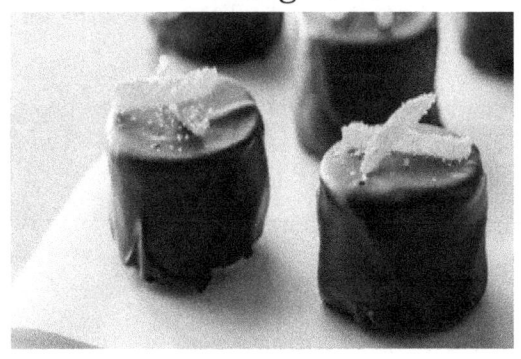

Preparation time: 20 minutes

Cooking time: 15 minutes

Servings: 6

Level of difficulty: Normal

Category: Healthy Fat

Ingredients:

- 10 ounces of coconut oil
- 4 tablespoons cocoa powder
- ¼ teaspoon blood orange extract
- stevia to taste

Directions:

1. Melt half of your coconut oil using a double boiler, and then add in your stevia and orange extract.
2. Get out candy molds, pouring the mixture into it. Fill each mold halfway, and then place in the fridge until they set.
3. Melt the other half of your coconut oil, stirring in your cocoa powder and stevia, ensuring that the mixture is smooth with no lumps.

4. Pour into your molds, filling them up all the way, and then allow it to set in the fridge before serving.

Nutrition:

Calories: 188 Protein: 1g

Fat: 21g Carbohydrates: 5g

169. Caramel Cones

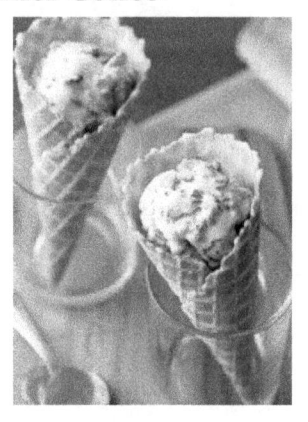

Preparation Time: 25 minutes

Cooking Time: 0 minutes

Servings: 6

Level of difficulty: Easy

Category: Healthy Fat

Ingredients:

- 2 tablespoons heavy whipping cream
- 2 tablespoons sour cream
- 1 tablespoon caramel sugar
- 1 teaspoon sea salt, fine
- 1/3 cup butter, grass-fed
- 1/3 cup coconut oil
- stevia to taste

Directions:

1. Soften your coconut oil and butter, mixing. Mix all fixings to form a batter, and then places them in molds. Top with a little salt, and keep refrigerated until serving.

Nutrition:

Calories: 251 Carbs: 29g

Fat: 13g Protein: 4g

170. Cinnamon Bites

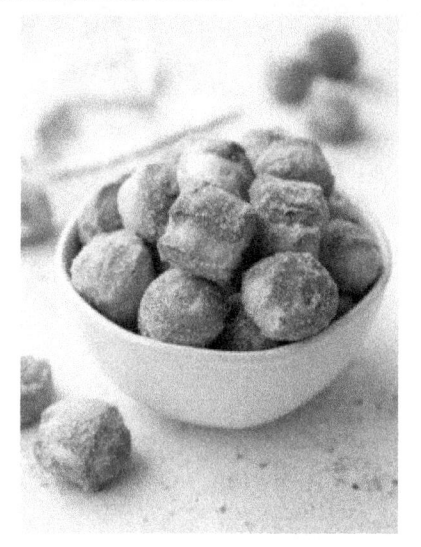

Preparation Time: 20 minutes

Cooking Time: 5 minutes

Servings: 6

Level of difficulty: Normal

Category: Healthy Fat

Ingredients:

- 1/8 teaspoon nutmeg

- 1 teaspoon vanilla extract
- ¼ teaspoon cinnamon
- 4 tablespoons coconut oil
- ½ cup butter, grass-fed
- 8 ounces cream cheese
- stevia to taste

Directions:

1. Soften your coconut oil and butter, mixing in your cream cheese. Add all of your remaining ingredients, and mix well. Pour into molds, and freeze until set.

Nutrition:

Calories: 180 Carbs: 29g

Fat: 6g Protein: 3g

171. Sweet Chai Bites

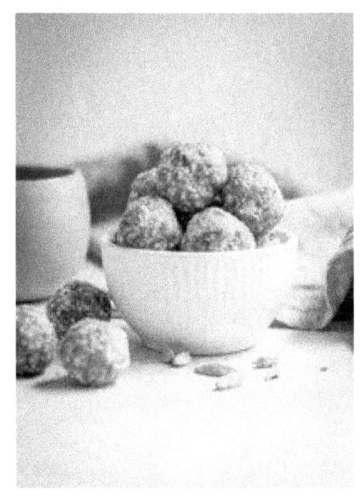

Preparation Time: 20 minutes

Cooking Time: 45 minutes

Servings: 6

Level of difficulty: Easy

Category: Healthy Fat

Ingredients:

- 1 cup cream cheese
- 1 cup of coconut oil
- 2 ounces butter, grass-fed
- 2 teaspoons ginger
- 2 teaspoons cardamom
- 1 teaspoon nutmeg
- 1 teaspoon cloves
- 1 teaspoon vanilla extract, pure
- 1 teaspoon Darjeeling black tea
- stevia to taste

Directions:

1. Melt your coconut oil and butter before adding in your black tea. Allow it to sit for one to two minutes.

2. Add in your cream cheese, removing your mixture from heat. Add in all of your spices, and stir to combine. Pour into molds, and freeze before serving.

Nutrition:

Calories: 178 Protein: 1g

Fat: 19g Carbs: 10g

172. Marinated Eggs

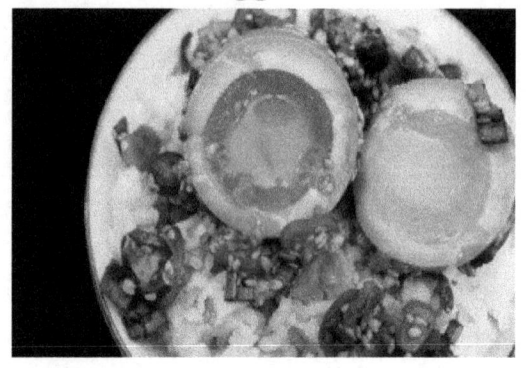

Preparation Time: 2 hours and 10 minutes

Cooking Time: 7 minutes

Servings: 4

Level of difficulty: Normal

Category: Lean

Ingredients:

- 6 eggs
- 1 and ¼ cups of water
- ¼ cup unsweetened rice vinegar
- 2 tablespoons coconut aminos
- Salt and black pepper to the taste
- 2 garlic cloves, minced
- 1 teaspoon stevia
- 4 ounces cream cheese
- 1 tablespoon chives, chopped

Directions:

1. Put the eggs in a pot, add water to cover, bring to a boil over medium heat, cover and cook for 7 minutes. Rinse eggs with cold water and leave them aside to cool down.
2. In a bowl, mix 1 cup water with coconut aminos, vinegar, stevia, and garlic and whisk well.
3. Put the eggs in this mix, cover with a kitchen towel, and leave them aside for 2 hours, rotating from time to time.
4. Peel eggs, cut in halves, and put egg yolks in a bowl. Add ¼ cup water, cream cheese, salt, pepper, and chives and stir well. Stuff egg whites with this mix and serve them.

Nutrition:

Calories: 289

Protein: 15.86 g

Fat: 22.62 g

Carbohydrates: 4.52 g

CHAPTER 12:

Desserts

173. Chocolate Bars

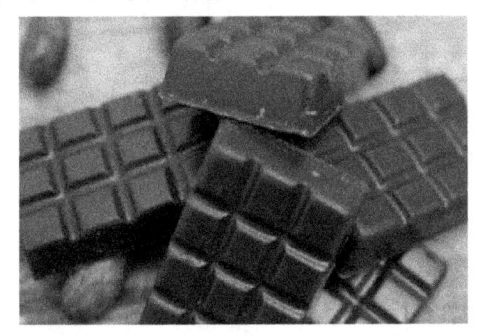

Preparation Time: 10 minutes

Cooking Time: 20 minutes

Servings: 16

Level of difficulty: Normal

Category: Healthy Fat

Ingredients:

- 15 oz cream cheese, softened
- 15 oz unsweetened dark chocolate
- 1 tsp vanilla - 10 drops liquid stevia

Directions:

1. Grease an 8-inch square dish and set aside. In a saucepan, dissolve chocolate over low heat. Add stevia and vanilla and stir well. Remove pan from heat and set aside. Add cream cheese into the blender and blend until smooth. Add melted chocolate mixture into the cream cheese and blend until just combined.
2. Transfer mixture into the prepared dish and spread evenly, and place in the refrigerator until firm. Slice and serve.

Nutrition: Calories: 230 Fat: 24 g

Carbs: 7.5 g Protein: 6 g

174. Blueberry Muffins

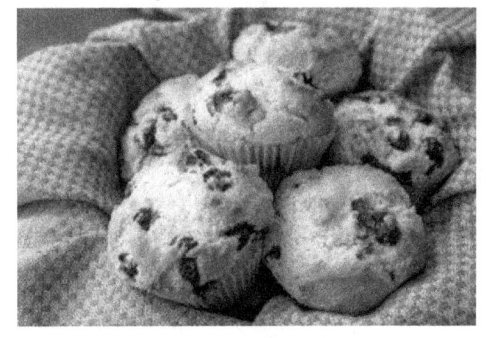

Preparation Time: 15 minutes

Cooking Time: 25 minutes

Servings: 12

Level of difficulty: Normal

Category: Healthy Fat

Ingredients:

- 2 eggs

- 1/2 cup fresh blueberries
- 1 cup heavy cream
- 2 cups almond flour
- 1/4 tsp lemon zest
- 1/2 tsp lemon extract
- 1 tsp baking powder
- 5 drops stevia
- 1/4 cup butter, melted

Directions:

1. Heat the cooker to 350 F. Line muffin tin with cupcake liners and set aside. Add eggs into the bowl and whisk until mix.
2. Add remaining ingredients and mix to combine, then pour the mixture into the prepared muffin tin and bake for 25 minutes. Serve and enjoy.

Nutrition:

Calories: 190

Fat: 17 g

Carbs: 5 g

Protein: 5 g

175. Chia Pudding

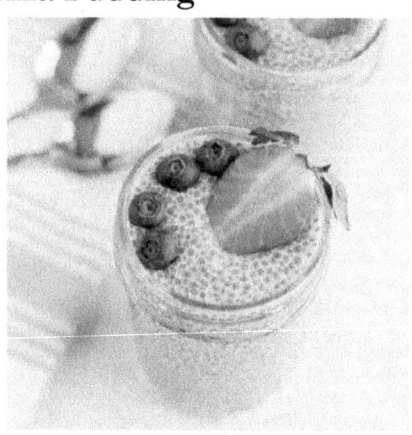

Preparation Time: 20 minutes

Cooking Time: 0 minutes

Servings: 2

Level of difficulty: Easy

Category: Healthy Fat

Ingredients:

- 4 tbsp chia seeds
- 1 cup unsweetened coconut milk
- 1/2 cup raspberries

Directions:

1. Add raspberry and coconut milk into a blender and blend until smooth. Pour mixture into the glass jar. Add chia seeds in a jar and stir well.
2. Seal the jar with a lid and shake well and place in the refrigerator for 3 hours. Serve chilled and enjoy.

Nutrition:

Calories: 360 Fat: 33 g Carbs: 13 g

Protein: 6 g

176. Avocado Pudding

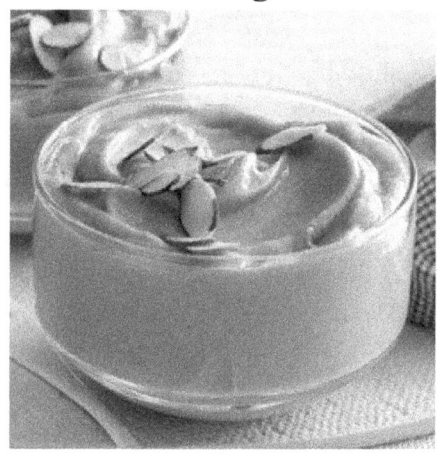

Preparation Time: 20 minutes

Cooking Time: 0 minutes

Servings: 8

Level of difficulty: Easy

Category: Green

Category: Healthy Fat

Ingredients:

- 2 ripe avocados, pitted and cut into pieces
- 1 tbsp fresh lime juice
- 14 oz coconut milk
- 2 tsp liquid stevia
- 2 tsp vanilla

Directions:

1. Inside the blender,

    Add all ingredients and blend until smooth. Serve immediately and enjoy.

Nutrition:

Calories: 317

Fat: 30 g

Carbs: 9 g

Protein: 3 g

177. Peanut Butter Coconut Popsicle

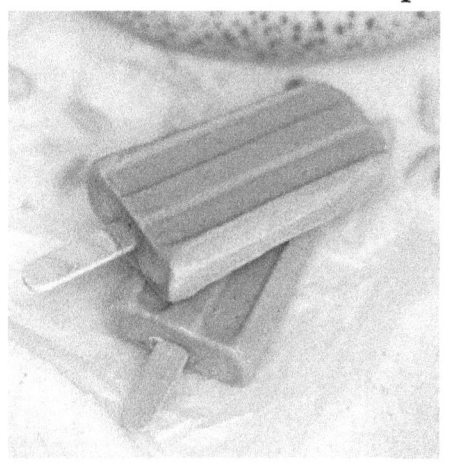

Preparation Time: 15 minutes

Cooking Time: 0 minutes

Servings: 12

Level of difficulty: Easy

Category: Healthy Fat

Ingredients:

- 1/2 cup peanut butter
- 1 tsp liquid stevia
- 2 cans unsweetened coconut milk

Directions:

1. In the blender, add all the listed ingredients and blend until smooth.

2. Pour mixture into the Popsicle molds and place in the freezer for 4 hours or until set. Serve!

Nutrition: Calories: 155 Fat: 15 g

Carbs: 4 g Protein: 3 g

178. Delicious Brownie Bites

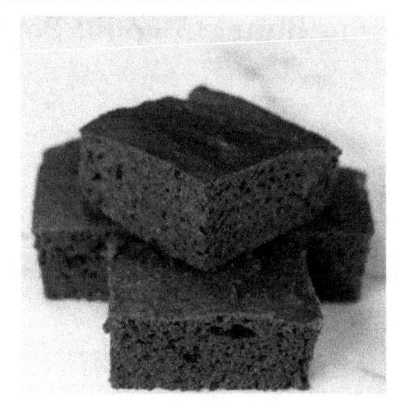

Preparation Time: 20 minutes

Cooking Time: 0 minutes

Servings: 13

Level of difficulty: Easy

Category: Healthy Fat

Ingredients:

- 1/4 cup unsweetened chocolate chips
- 1/4 cup unsweetened cocoa powder
- 1 cup pecans, chopped
- 1/2 cup almond butter
- 1/2 tsp vanilla - 1/8 tsp pink salt
- 1/4 cup monk fruit sweetener

Directions:

1. Add pecans, sweetener, vanilla, almond butter, cocoa powder, and salt into the food processor and process until well combined. Transfer brownie mixture into the large bowl.

2. Add chocolate chips and fold well. Make small round shape balls from brownie mixture and place onto a baking tray. Place in the freezer for 20 minutes. Serve and enjoy.

Nutrition: Calories: 108 Fat: 9 g

Carbs: 4 g Protein: 2 g

179. Pumpkin Balls

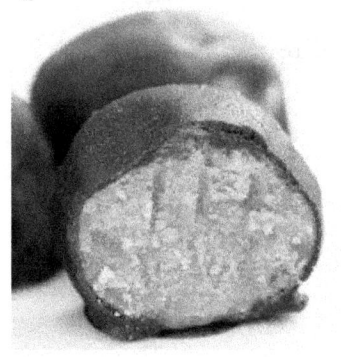

Preparation Time: 15 minutes

Cooking Time: 0 minutes

Servings: 18

Level of difficulty: Easy

Category: Green

Ingredients: 1 cup almond butter

- 5 drops liquid stevia
- 2 tbsp coconut flour

- 2 tbsp pumpkin puree
- 1 tsp pumpkin pie spice

Directions:

1. Mix pumpkin puree in a large bowl and almond butter until well combined. Add liquid stevia, pumpkin pie spice, and coconut flour and mix well.
2. Make small balls from the mixture and place onto a baking tray in the freezer for 1 hour. Serve and enjoy.

Nutrition: Calories: 96 Fat: 8 g

Carbs: 4 g Protein: 2 g

180. Smooth Peanut Butter Cream

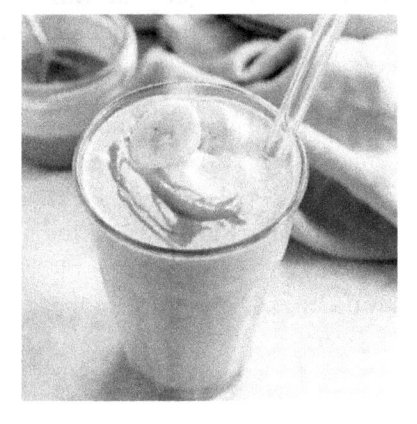

Preparation Time: 10 minutes

Cooking Time: 0 minutes

Servings: 8

Level of difficulty: Easy

Category: Healthy Fat

Ingredients:

- 1/4 cup peanut butter

- 4 overripe bananas, chopped
- 1/3 cup cocoa powder
- 1/4 tsp vanilla extract - 1/8 tsp salt

Directions:

1. In the blender, add all the listed ingredients and blend until smooth. Serve immediately and enjoy.

Nutrition: Calories: 101 Fat: 5 g

Carbs: 14 g Protein: 3 g

181. Vanilla Avocado Popsicles

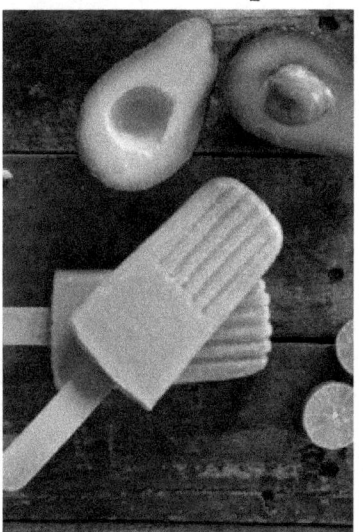

Preparation Time: 20 minutes

Cooking Time: 0 minutes

Servings: 6

Level of difficulty: Easy

Category: Healthy Fat

Ingredients:

- 2 avocadoes

- 1 tsp vanilla
- 1 cup almond milk
- 1 tsp liquid stevia
- 1/2 cup unsweetened cocoa powder

Directions:

1. In the blender, add all the listed ingredients and blend smoothly. Pour blended mixture into the Popsicle molds and place in the freezer until set. Serve and enjoy.

Nutrition:

Calories: 130

Fat: 12 g

Carbs: 7 g

Protein: 3 g

182. Chocolate Popsicle

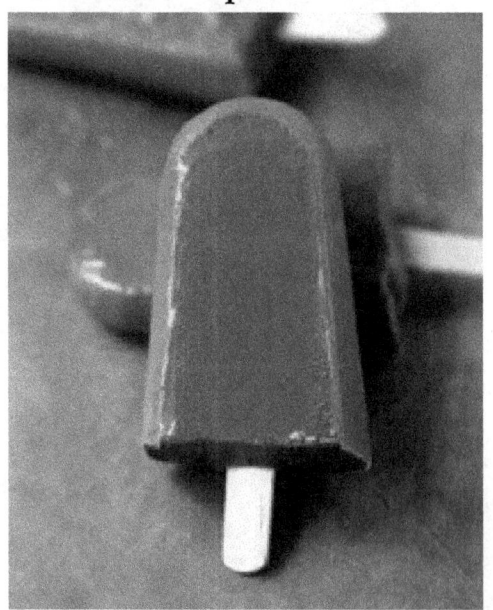

Preparation Time: 20 minutes

Cooking Time: 10 minutes

Servings: 6

Level of difficulty: Easy

Category: Healthy Fat

Ingredients:

- 4 oz unsweetened chocolate, chopped
- 6 drops liquid stevia
- 1 1/2 cups heavy cream

Directions:

1. Add heavy cream into the microwave-safe bowl and microwave until it just begins the boiling. Add chocolate into the heavy cream and set aside for 5 minutes.
2. Add liquid stevia into the heavy cream mixture and stir until chocolate is melted. Pour mixture into the Popsicle molds and place in freezer for 4 hours or until set. Serve and enjoy.

Nutrition:

Calories: 198

Fat: 21 g

Carbs: 6 g

Protein: 3 g

183. Raspberry Ice Cream

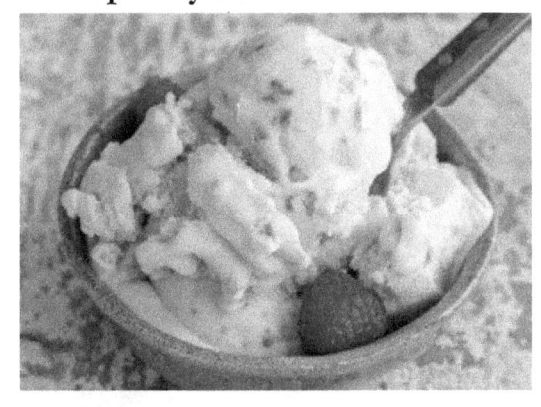

Preparation Time: 10 minutes

Cooking Time: 0 minutes

Servings: 2

Level of difficulty: Easy

Category: Healthy Fat

Ingredients:

- 1 cup frozen raspberries
- 1/2 cup heavy cream
- 1/8 tsp stevia powder

Directions:

1. Blend all the listed fixings in a blender until smooth. Serve immediately and enjoy.

Nutrition:

Calories: 144

Fat: 11 g

Carbs: 10 g

Protein: 2 g

184. Chocolate Frosty

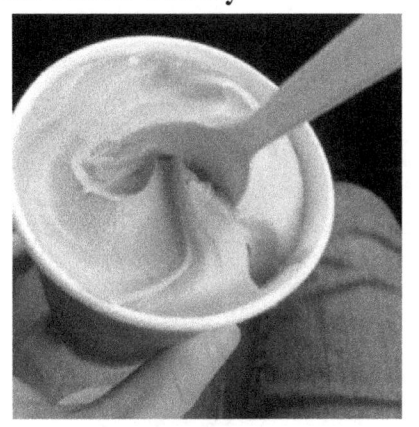

Preparation Time: 20 minutes

Cooking Time: 0 minutes

Servings: 4

Level of difficulty: Easy

Category: Healthy Fat

Ingredients:

- 2 tbsp unsweetened cocoa powder
- 1 cup heavy whipping cream
- 1 tbsp almond butter
- 5 drops liquid stevia - 1 tsp vanilla

Directions:

1. Add cream into the medium bowl and beat using the hand mixer for 5 minutes. Add remaining ingredients and blend until thick cream forms.
2. Pour in serving bowls and place them in the freezer for 30 minutes. Serve and enjoy.

Nutrition: Calories: 137 Fat: 13 g

Carbs: 3 g Protein: 2 g

185. Chocolate Almond Butter Brownie

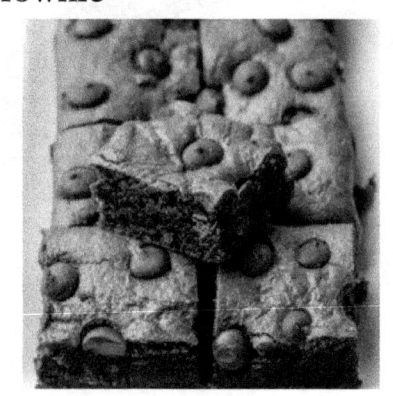

Preparation Time: 10 minutes

Cooking Time: 16 minutes

Servings: 4

Level of difficulty: Normal

Category: Healthy Fat

Ingredients:

- 1 cup bananas, overripe
- 1/2 cup almond butter, melted
- 1 scoop protein powder
- 2 tbsp unsweetened cocoa powder

Directions:

1. Warm air fryer to 325 F. Grease air fryer baking pan and set aside. Blend all fixings in a blender until smooth.
2. Pour batter into the prepared pan and place in the air fryer basket, and cook for 16 minutes. Serve and enjoy.

Nutrition: Calories: 82 Fat: 2 g

Carbs: 11 g Protein: 7 g

186. Peanut Butter Fudge

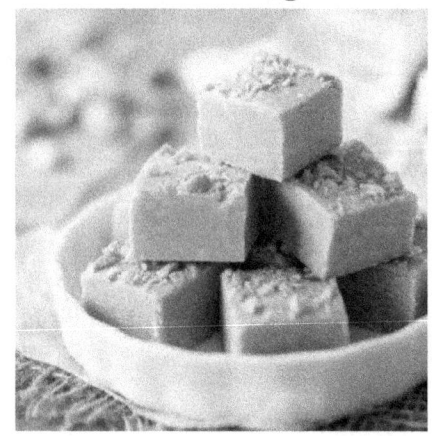

Preparation Time: 10 minutes

Cooking Time: 10 minutes

Servings: 20

Level of difficulty: Normal

Category: Healthy Fat

Ingredients:

- 1/4 cup almonds, toasted and chopped
- 12 oz smooth peanut butter
- 15 drops liquid stevia
- 3 tbsp coconut oil
- 4 tbsp coconut cream
- Pinch of salt

Directions:

1. Line baking tray with parchment paper. Dissolve coconut oil in a pan over low heat. Add peanut butter, coconut cream, stevia, and salt in a saucepan. Stir well.

2. Pour fudge mixture into the prepared baking tray and sprinkle chopped almonds on top. Place the tray in the refrigerator for 1 hour or until set. Slice and serve.

Nutrition:

Calories: 131

Fat: 12 g

Carbs: 4 g

CHAPTER 13:

Smoothies

187. Creamy Raspberry Pomegranate Smoothie

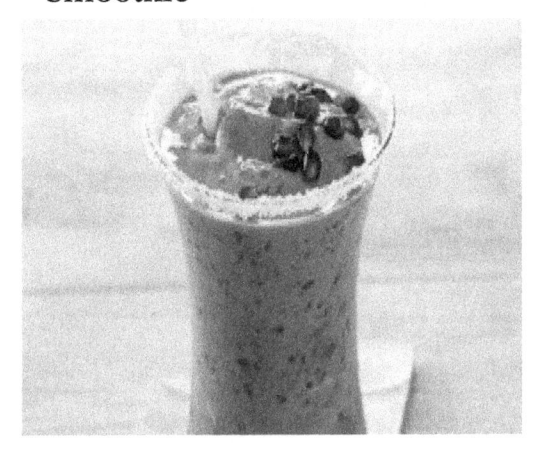

Preparation Time: 5 minutes

Cooking Time: 0 minutes

Level of difficulty: Easy

Servings: 1

Category: Green

Ingredients:

- 1½ cups pomegranate juice
- ½ cup unsweetened coconut milk
- 1 scoop vanilla protein powder
- 2 packed cups fresh baby spinach
- 1 cup frozen raspberries
- 1 frozen banana
- 1 to 2 tablespoons freshly compressed lemon juice

Directions:

1. In a blender, combine the pomegranate juice and coconut milk. Add the protein powder and spinach. Give these a whirl to break down the spinach.
2. Add the raspberries, banana, and lemon juice, then top it off with ice. Blend until smooth and frothy.

Nutrition:

Calories: 303

fat: 3g

Carbs: 0g

Protein: 15g

188. Avocado Kale Smoothie

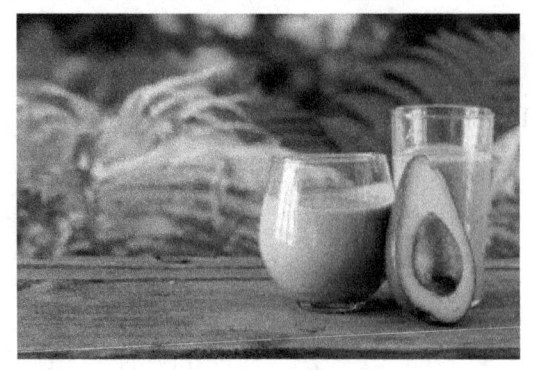

Preparation Time: 5 minutes

Cooking Time: 0 minutes

Servings: 3

Level of difficulty: Easy

Category: Green/Healthy Fat

Ingredients:

- 1 cup of water
- ½ Seville orange, peeled
- 1 avocado
- 1 cucumber, peeled
- 1 cup kale
- 1 cup of ice cubes

Directions:

1. Toss all your ingredients into your blender, then process till smooth and creamy. Serve immediately and enjoy.

Nutrition:

Calories: 160 Fat: 13.3g

Carbs: 11.6g

Protein: 2.4g

189. Apple Kale Cucumber Smoothie

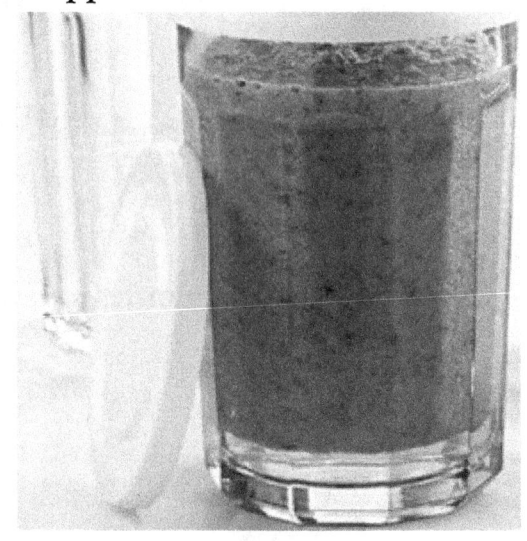

Preparation Time: 5 minutes

Cooking Time: 0 minutes

Servings: 1

Level of difficulty: Easy

Category: Green

Ingredients:

- ¾ cup of water
- ½ green apple, diced
- ¾ cup kale
- ½ cucumber

Directions:

1. Toss all your ingredients into your blender, then process till smooth and creamy. Serve immediately and enjoy.

Nutrition:

Calories: 86 Fat: 0.5g

Carbs: 21.7g Protein: 1.9g

190. Refreshing Cucumber Smoothie

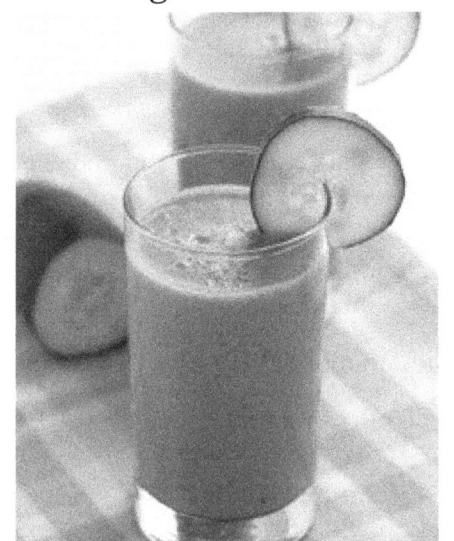

Preparation Time: 5 minutes

Cooking Time: 0 minutes

Servings: 2

Level of difficulty: Easy

Category: Green

Ingredients:

- 1 cup of ice cubes
- 20 drops liquid stevia
- 2 fresh lime, peeled and halved
- 1 tsp lime zest, grated
- 1 cucumber, chopped
- 1 avocado, pitted and peeled
- 2 cups kale
- 1 tbsp creamed coconut
- ¾ cup of coconut water

Directions:

1. Toss all your ingredients into your blender, then process till smooth and creamy. Serve immediately and enjoy.

Nutrition: Calories: 313 Fat: 25.1g

Carbs: 24.7g Protein: 4.9g

191. Cauliflower Veggie Smoothie

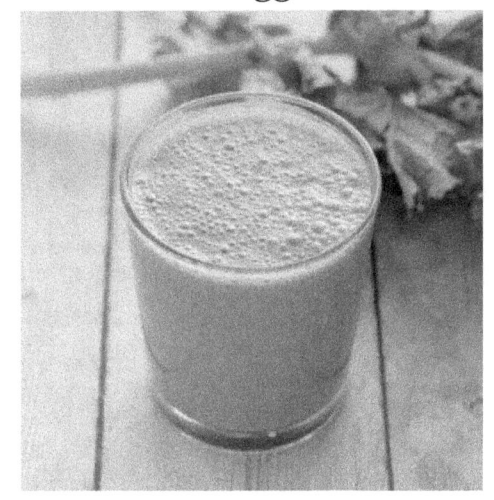

Preparation Time: 5 minutes

Cooking Time: 5 minutes

Servings: 4

Level of difficulty: Easy

Category: Green

Ingredients:

- 1 zucchini, peeled and chopped
- 1 Seville orange, peeled
- 1 apple, diced - 1 banana
- 1 cup kale - ½ cup cauliflower

Directions:

1. Toss all your ingredients into your blender, then process till smooth and creamy. Serve immediately and enjoy.

Nutrition: Calories: 71 Fat: 0.3g

Carbs: 18.3g Protein: 1.3g

192. Soursop Smoothie

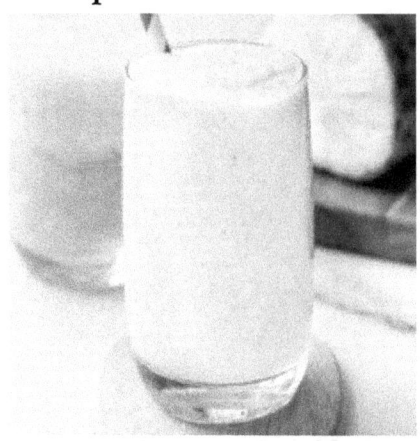

Preparation Time: 5 minutes

Cooking Time: 0 minutes

Servings: 2

Level of difficulty: Easy

Category: Green

Ingredients:

- 3 quartered frozen Burro Bananas
- 1-1/2 cups of Homemade Coconut Milk
- 1/4 cup of Walnuts
- 1 teaspoon of Sea Moss Gel
- 1 teaspoon of Ground Ginger
- 1 teaspoon of Soursop Leaf Powder
- 1 handful of kale

Directions:

1. Prepare and put all ingredients in a blender or a food processor. Blend it well until you reach a smooth consistency. Serve and enjoy your Soursop Smoothie!

Nutrition: Calories: 213 Fat: 3.1g

Carbs: 6g Protein: 8g

193. Tiramisu Shake

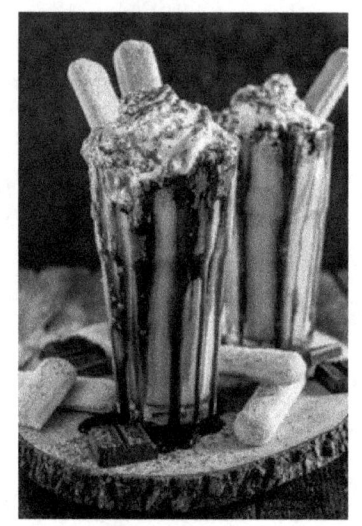

Preparation time: 5 minutes

Cooking time: 0 minutes

Servings: 1

Level of difficulty: Easy

Category: Healthy Fat

Ingredients:

- 1 packet Medifast cappuccino mix

- 1 tablespoon sugar-free chocolate syrup
- ½ cup of water - ½ cup ice, crushed

Directions:

1. In a small blender, place all ingredients and pulse until smooth and creamy. Transfer the shake into a serving glass and serve immediately.

Nutrition: Calories: 107 Fat: 0g

Carbohydrates: 15g Protein: 14g

194. Vanilla Shake

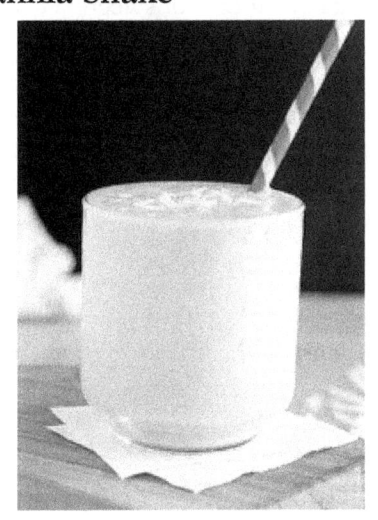

Preparation time: 5 minutes

Cooking time: 0 minutes

Servings: 1

Level of difficulty: Easy

Category: Healthy Fat

Ingredients:

- ½ packet Lean and Green Vanilla Shake Fueling

- ½ packet Optavia Gingerbread Fueling
- ½ cup unsweetened almond milk
- ½ cup of water - 8 ice cubes

Directions:

1. In a small blender, place all ingredients and pulse until smooth. Transfer the smoothie into a serving glass and serve immediately.

Nutrition: Calories: 130 Fat: 3.3g

Carbohydrates: 15g Protein: 13g

195. Shamrock Shake

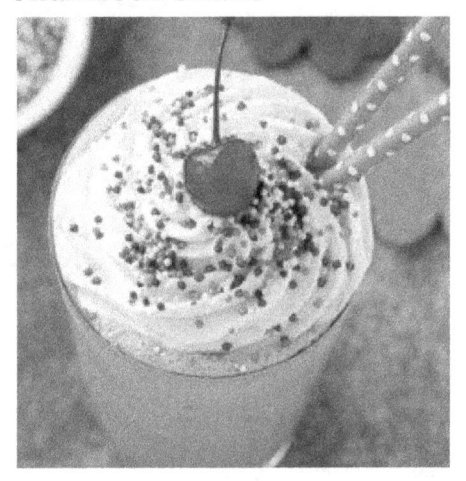

Preparation time: 5 minutes

Cooking time: 0 minutes

Servings: 1

Level of difficulty: Easy

Category: Healthy Fat

Ingredients:

- 1 packet Medifast Vanilla Shake

- 6 ounces unsweetened almond milk
- ¼ teaspoon peppermint extract
- 1-2 drops green food coloring
- 1 cup of ice cubes

Directions:

1. In a small blender, place all ingredients and pulse until smooth. Transfer the smoothie into a serving glass and serve immediately.

Nutrition:

Calories: 120

Fat: 3.9g

Carbohydrates: 13.5g

Protein: 11.7g

196. Coconut Smoothie

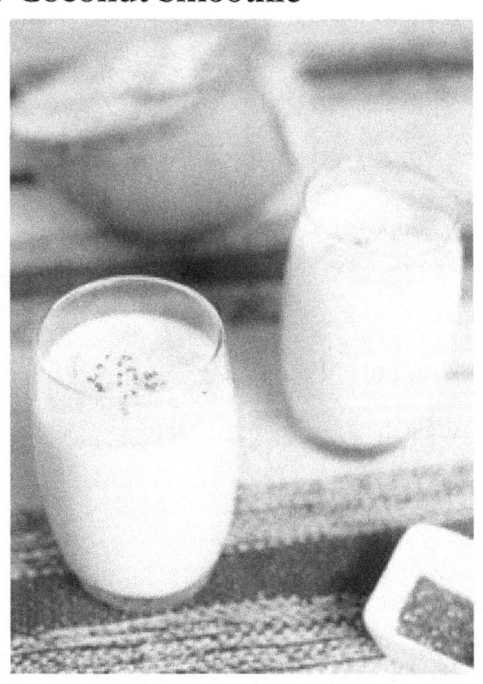

Preparation time: 5 minutes

Cooking time: 0 minutes

Servings: 1

Level of difficulty: Easy

Category: Healthy Fat

Ingredients:

- 1 sachet Lean and Green Essential Creamy Vanilla Shake
- 6 ounces unsweetened almond milk
- 6 ounces diet ginger ale
- 2 tablespoons unsweetened coconut, shredded
- ¼ teaspoon rum extract
- ½ cup ice

Directions:

1. In a small blender, place all ingredients and pulse until smooth. Transfer the smoothie into a serving glass and serve immediately.

Nutrition:

Calories: 120

Fat: 6.2g

Carbohydrates: 15.9g

Protein: 15g

197. Vanilla Frappe

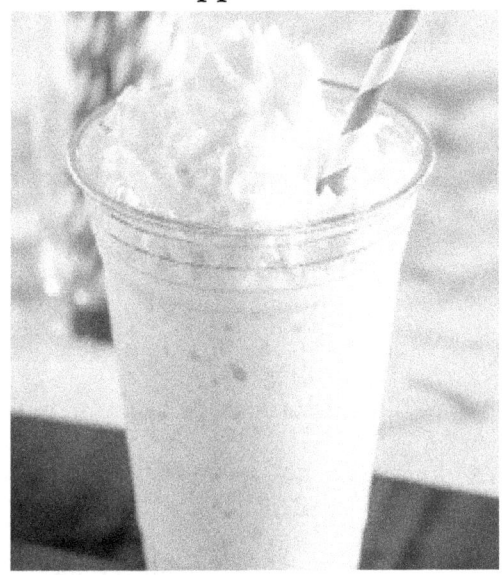

Preparation time: 5 minutes

Cooking time: 0 minutes

Servings: 1

Level of difficulty: Easy

Category: Healthy Fat

Ingredients:

- 1 sachet Lean and Green Essential Vanilla Shake
- 8 ounces unsweetened almond milk
- ½ cup ice
- 1 tablespoon whipped topping

Directions:

1. In a blender, add the Vanilla Shake sachet, almond milk, and ice and pulse until smooth. Transfer the mixture into a glass and top with whipped topping. Serve immediately.

Nutrition:

Calories: 155

Fat: 4.4g

Carbohydrates: 15.2g

Protein: 15g

198. Pumpkin Frappe

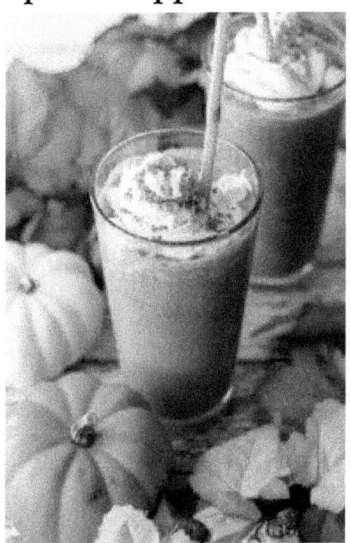

Preparation time: 5 minutes

Cooking time: 0 minutes

Servings: 1

Level of difficulty: Easy

Category: Healthy Fat

Ingredients:

- 1 sachet Lean and Green Essential Spiced Gingerbread
- 4 ounces strong brewed coffee
- 4 ounces unsweetened almond milk

- 1/8 teaspoon pumpkin pie spice
- ½ cup ice
- 1 tablespoon whipped topping

Directions:

1. In a blender, add the Spiced Gingerbread sachet, coffee, almond milk, pumpkin pie spice, and ice and pulse until smooth. Transfer the mixture into a glass and top with whipped topping. Serve immediately.

Nutrition:

Calories: 138

Fat: 4.8g

Carbohydrates: 16.4g

Protein: 11.7g

199. Chocolate Frappe

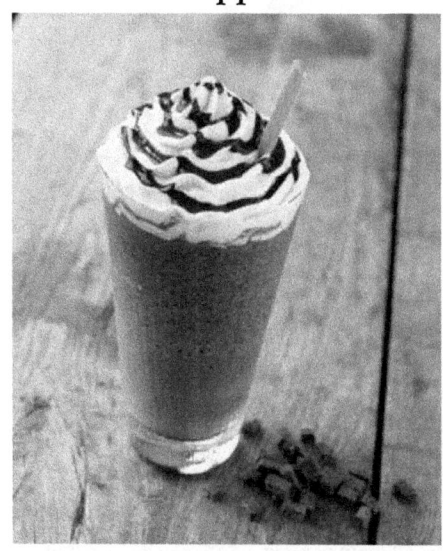

Preparation time: 5 minutes

Cooking time: 0 minutes

Servings: 1

Level of difficulty: Easy

Category: Healthy Fat

Ingredients:

- 1 sachet Lean and Green Essential Frosty Mint Chocolate Soft Serve Treat
- 4 ounces strong brewed coffee
- 4 ounces unsweetened almond milk
- 1½ tablespoons sugar-free chocolate syrup, divided
- ¼ teaspoon peppermint extract
- ½ cup ice
- 1 tablespoon whipped topping

Directions:

1. In a blender, add the Chocolate sachet, coffee, almond milk, 1 tablespoon of chocolate syrup, peppermint extract, and ice and pulse until smooth.
2. Transfer the mixture into a glass and top with whipped topping. Drizzle with remaining chocolate syrup and serve immediately.

Nutrition:

Calories: 148

Fat: 4.8g

Carbohydrates: 18g

Protein: 11.7g

200. Peppermint Mocha Shake

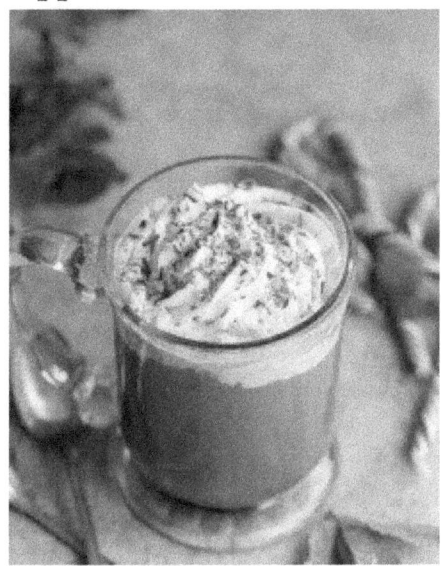

Preparation time: 5 minutes

Cooking time: 0 minutes

Servings: 1

Level of difficulty: Easy

Category: Healthy Fat

Ingredients:

- 1 sachet Lean and Green Essential Velvety Hot Chocolate
- 6 ounces freshly brewed coffee
- ¼ cup warm unsweetened almond milk
- ¼ teaspoon peppermint extract
- One tablespoon whipped topping
- Pinch of ground cinnamon

Directions:

1. In a serving mug, place the Hot Chocolate sachet, coffee, almond milk, and peppermint extract and stir until well blended.
2. Top the hot chocolate with whipped topping and sprinkle with cinnamon. Serve immediately.

Nutrition:

Calories: 133

Fat: 1.1g

Carbohydrates: 15.2g

Protein: 14.6g

LEAN AND GREEN DIET COOKBOOK:

CHAPTER 14:

Optavia 28 Days Meal Plan and Shopping List

201. Shopping List Week 1

Agave, Allspice, amaranth, arborio rice, arrowroot powder, avocado, baby bok choy baby peas, baby spinach, baking powder, banana, barley, bay leaf, black beans, black-eyed peas, Blue cheese dressing, blueberries, braggs liquid aminos, brown sugar, Buns, Burro Bananas, butter, buttermilk cheddar herb biscuit, button mushrooms, carrots, cherry tomatoes, chicken breast, chickpeas, chili powder, chili sauce, cilantro, coconut, coconut flour, coconut milk, coconut oil, cooking spray, cremini mushrooms, cucumber, dill pickle, dried basil, dried marjoram leaves, dried oregano, dried red lentils, dried thyme leaves, eggs, fennel bulb, garlic, garlic powder, ginger, grapeseed oil, Greek yogurt, green apple, green chili, ground cinnamon, ground cumin, Ground Ginger, ground nutmeg, honey, hulled barley, jalapeno, kale, kidney beans, Lean Chicken, lean ground beef, leek, lemon, Lettuce, Lime, liquid stevia, low-fat cheddar cheese, maple syrup, Medifast cappuccino mix, milk mozzarella cheese, nutmeg, oat bran/oat flour (gluten-free), olive oil, olives, onion powder, Lean and Green select, orange, oregano, parsley, pear, pomegranate, raisins, Ranch dressing, raspberries, red bell pepper, red onion, salmon fillets, salt, scallions, sea moss gel, sea salt, sesame seeds, short-grain brown rice, Soursop Leaf Powder, soy sauce, spelt flour, squash, sugar, sugar-free chocolate syrup, sweet potato, teff flour, tempeh, tofu, tomato paste, tomato sauce, turkey, vanilla extract, vanilla paste, vanilla protein powder, Walnuts, white champignons, white whole-wheat flour, whole-milk ricotta cheese, wild rice, Worcestershire sauce, yellow mustard, yellow onion, and zucchinis.

Meal Plan Week 1

Day	Breakfast	Lunch	Dinner	Snacks/Sides	Smoothies
1	Alkaline Blueberry Spelt Cake	Baked Ricotta with Pears	Bok Choy with Tofu Stir Fry	Bacon Cheeseburger	Creamy Raspberry Pomegranate Smoothie
2	Alkaline Blueberry Muffins	Herbed Wild Rice	Three-Bean Medley	Cheeseburger Pie	Avocado Kale Smoothie
3	Crunchy Quinoa Meal	Buffalo Chicken Sliders	Herbed Garlic Black Beans	Personal Pizza Biscuit	Apple Kale Cucumber Smoothie
4	Coconut Pancakes	High Protein Chicken Meatballs	Quinoa with Vegetables	Chicken and Mushroom	Refreshing Cucumber Smoothie
5	Quinoa Porridge	Barley Risotto	Pan-Fried Salmon	Chicken Enchilada Bake	Cauliflower Veggie Smoothie
6	Amaranth Porridge	Risotto with Green Beans, Sweet Potatoes, and Peas	Mediterranean Chickpea Salad	Jalapeno Lentil (Chickpea) Burgers + Avocado Mango Pico	Soursop Smoothie
7	Banana Barley Porridge	Maple Lemon Tempeh Cubes	Zucchini Salmon Salad	Grandma Rice	Tiramisu Shake

Shopping List Week 2

Almond, almond butter, avocados, baking powder, balsamic vinegar, banana, basil leaves, bay leaf, blood orange extract, brewed coffee, broccoli, brown mushrooms, Butter grass-fed, caramel sugar, carrot, cayenne pepper, celery stalk, cheddar cheese, cherry tomatoes, chia seeds, chicken bouillon cubes, chicken breasts, chili powder, chives, cilantro, cinnamon, cocoa powder, coconut, coconut butter, coconut flakes, coconut flour, cod, coriander, cream cheese, cumin, diet ginger ale, dried basil, dried dill, dry steak seasonings, dry white wine, eggs, fennel bulb, fennel seeds, Flax Seeds, garlic, garlic powder, ginger, ginger powder, green chilies, green food coloring, green plantain, ground chicken, ground cinnamon, ground cumin, ground turmeric, heavy whipping cream, hemp seed, Italian seasoning, jackfruit, jalapeño peppers, lean beef, lean lamb, lean pork, lemon, lime, liquid stevia, Medifast Vanilla Shake, millet, mushroom, olive oil, onion, onion powder, Lean and Green Essential Frosty Mint Chocolate Soft Serve Treat, Lean and Green Essential Spiced Gingerbread, Lean and Green Essential Vanilla Shake, Lean and Green essential Velvety Hot Chocolate, Lean and Green Gingerbread Fueling, Lean and Green Vanilla Shake Fueling, orange, oregano, parmesan cheese, parsley, pepper, peppermint extract, potatoes, pumpkin, pumpkin pie spice, red bell peppers, red onion, rum extract, salmon fillets, salt, skinless chicken thighs, sour cream, spinach, stevia, strawberries, sugar-free chocolate syrup, sweet paprika, thyme, thyme sprig tomato, tomato paste, unsweetened almond milk, vanilla extract, walnut butter, wild rice, yellow onion, and zucchinis.

Meal Plan Week 2

Day	Breakfast	Lunch	Dinner	Snacks/Sides	Smoothies
8	Zucchini Muffins	Greek Roasted Fish	Chicken Broccoli Salad with Avocado Dressing	Bake Beef Zucchini	Vanilla Shake
9	Millet Porridge	Oregano Pork Mix	Balsamic Beef and Mushroom Mix	Lamb Stuffed Avocado	Shamrock Shake
10	Jackfruit Vegetable Fry	Simple Beef Roast	Garlicky Tomato Chicken Casserole	Sweet Almond Bites	Coconut Smoothie
11	Zucchini Pancakes	Pork & Peppers Chili	Fennel Wild Rice Risotto	Strawberry Cheesecake Minis	Vanilla Frappe
12	Squash Hash	Chicken Breast Soup	Garlic Chicken Balls	Cocoa Brownies	Pumpkin Frappe
13	Hemp Seed Porridge	Tomato Fish Bake	Sliced Steak with Canadian Crust	Chocolate Orange Bites	Chocolate Frappe
14	Pumpkin Spice Quinoa	Warm Chorizo Chickpea Salad	Chicken Sancho	Caramel Cones	Peppermint Mocha Shake

Shopping List Week 3

Almond flour, almonds, apple, apple cider vinegar, assorted seeds, avocado, baby spinach, bacon, baking powder, banana, Black beans, black chili pepper, black pepper, bone-free pork chops, broccoli, broccoli blossoms, Burro Bananas, canned pumpkin, cardamom, carrots, cauliflower, cayenne chili pepper, cheddar cheese, Cheese (Nonfat), chicken sausage, Chinese plum sauce, chipotle chili pepper, chipotle chilies in adobo sauce, chives, chocolate chips, cilantro leaves, cinnamon, cloves, cocoa powder, coconut, coconut aminos, coconut flakes, coconut flour, coconut oil, cornstarch, cream cheese, cucumber, cumin, Darjeeling black tea, Dijon mustard, dried cherries, dried thyme, egg noodles, eggs, erythritol, extra-virgin olive oil, fat-cut pork tenderloin, fat-free gravy beef jar, fresh pea pods, garlic, garlic powder, ginger, goat cheese, grass-fed butter, green apple, ground cinnamon, ground flaxseed, Ground Ginger, honey, Hot sauce, kale, Kosher salt, lamb chops, lasagna noodles, lean beef, lean ground beef, leg of lamb, lemon, lime, liquid stevia, low carb ketchup, low-fat sour cream, mango, maple syrup, mayonnaise light, Medifast cappuccino mix, mild salsa, mini peppers, molasses, nutmeg, oat flour, onion, onion powder, orange, oregano, peanut oil, peanuts, pickles, pomegranate juice, potatoes, raspberries, red pepper flakes, red vinegar, regular breadcrumbs, rice vinegar, ricotta cheese, rolled oats, rosemary leaves, sage, scallions, Sea Moss Gel, sea salt, sesame oil, sesame seeds, sirloin fillet, skinless chicken breast, Soursop Leaf Powder, soy milk, soy sauce, spinach, steel cut oats, sugar-free chocolate syrup, sweet paprika, thyme, tomato sauce, unsweetened coconut milk, vanilla extract, vanilla protein powder, Walnuts, white mushrooms, white wine, whole grain tortilla, Whole wheat noodles, whole-wheat hamburger buns, Worcestershire sauce, xylitol, yellow mustard, and zucchini.

Meal Plan Week 3

Day	Breakfast	Lunch	Dinner	Snacks/Sides	Smoothies
15	Chocolate Cherry Crunch Granola	Mexican Chicken in Orange Juice	Beef and Chicken Sausage-Stuffed Mini Peppers	Cinnamon Bites	Creamy Raspberry Pomegranate Smoothie
16	Mango Coconut Oatmeal	Adobo Sirloin	Grilled Rosemary Lamb Chops	Sweet Chai Bites	Avocado Kale Smoothie
17	Scrambled Eggs with Soy Sauce and Broccoli Slaw	Beef Stroganoff	Honey-Mustard Leg of Lamb	Marinated Eggs	Apple Kale Cucumber Smoothie
18	Tasty Breakfast Donuts	Beef Lo Mein	Pork Chops Braised with Oranges	Caramelized Onion Quesadilla	Refreshing Cucumber Smoothie
19	Cheesy Spicy Bacon Bowls	Beef Lasagna	Plum Sauce-Glazed Pork Chops	Roasted Garlic Potatoes	Cauliflower Veggie Smoothie
20	Goat Cheese Zucchini Kale Quiche	Teriyaki Sirloin Steaks	Dijon and Sage-Coated Pork Tenderloin	Asian Noodle Salad	Soursop Smoothie
21	Ricotta Ramekins	Salisbury Steak	Smothered Cajun Pork Chops with Tomatoes	Protein Pumpkin Spiced Donuts	Tiramisu Shake

Shopping List Week 4

Agave syrup, almond flour, almond milk, almonds, apple cider vinegar, artichokes, asparagus, avocado oil, bacon, blueberries, brewed coffee, broccoli, Brussels sprouts, cabbage, Cajun seasoning, calamari tubes, cane sugar or agave nectar carrots, cashews, catfish fillets, cauliflower florets, celery, Cheddar cheese, chia seeds, chicken breast, chicken seasoning, chili flakes, chocolate, cilantro, club soda, coconut, coconut cream, coconut flour, coconut milk, coconut oil, cod fillets, Cornmeal, cornstarch, curry powder, diet ginger ale, dill pickle, dried basil, dried herbs, dried oregano, dried thyme, eggs, fennel heads, fish sauce, flour, fresh basil, fresh dill, fresh tuna, garlic, garlic powder, ginger, Greek yogurt, green beans, green food coloring, ground black pepper, ground bourbon vanilla, ground cinnamon, ground turmeric, half and half, hazelnuts, heavy cream, honey, kosher salt, lavender, lemon, lemon pepper seasoning, low carb bread, low-fat whipping cream, maple syrup, mayonnaise, Medifast Vanilla Shake, mozzarella cheese ,nutmeg, nutritional yeast, oatmeal flour, oil spray, olive oil, onion, onion powder, Lean and Green Essential Frosty Mint Chocolate Soft Serve Treat, Lean and Green Essential Spiced Gingerbread, Lean and Green Essential Vanilla Shake, Lean and Green Essential Velvety Hot Chocolate, Lean and Green Gingerbread Fueling, Lean and Green Vanilla Shake Fueling, orange, oregano, organic quark, panko breadcrumbs, paprika, parmesan cheese, parsley, peanut butter, peppermint extract, pomegranate, Portobello mushroom hats, potatoes, powdered sugar, pumpkin pie spice, raw shrimp, red pepper, red pepper flakes, rice vinegar, rum extract, salmon fillets, salsa, sea scallops, serrano chili, smoked eel, snow peas, soy yogurt, spelled flour, spinach, spring onions, spring roll wrappers, sriracha, stevia liquid, sugar-free chocolate syrup, sunflower seeds, sweet chili sauce, thyme, tomato paste, tomatoes, unsweetened almond milk, walnuts, White pepper, whole chicken, whole wheat breadcrumbs, yogurt, and zucchinis.

Meal Plan Week 4

Day	Breakfast	Lunch	Dinner	Snacks/Sides	Smoothies
22	Chicken Lo Mein	Pesto Zucchini Noodles	Sriracha & Honey Tossed Calamari	Coconut Fat Bombs	Vanilla Shake
23	Pancakes with Berries	Baked Cod & Vegetables	Southern Style Catfish with Green Beans	Easy One-Pot Vegan Marinara	Shamrock Shake
24	Omelet À La Margherita	Chicken Zucchini Noodles	Roasted Salmon with Fennel Salad	Sunflower Parmesan Cheese	Coconut Smoothie
25	Coconut Chia Pudding with Berries	Chicken Casserole	Catfish with Cajun Seasoning	Spicy Zucchini Slices	Vanilla Frappe
26	Eel on Scrambled Eggs and Bread	Brussels Sprout Curry	Garlic-Lime Shrimp Kebabs	Cheddar Portobello Mushrooms	Pumpkin Frappe
27	Chia Seed Gel with Pomegranate and Nuts	Shrimp Spring Rolls	Healthy Tun Patties	Salty Lemon Artichokes	Chocolate Frappe
28	Lavender Blueberry Chia Seed Pudding	Scallops with Tomato Cream Sauce	Breaded Air Fried Shrimp with Bang-Bang Sauce	Cheddar Potato Gratin	Peppermint Mocha Shake

Conclusion

You had reached the end of this cookbook. You now know a lot about the Optavia Diet and even about the recommended recipes for this diet. Now, let's wrapped this up with the frequently asked question (FAQ):

How Much Weight, On Average, You Can Lose with The Optimal Weight Plan 5 And 1?

On the Optimal weight plan 5 and 1, the average weight shed is around 12 pounds. Clients have an average of 12 weeks of weight loss. Lean and Green suggests you notify your medical professional before beginning a weight-reduction program.

Should A Person Go in The Optimal Weight 5 And 1 Plan If He Didn't Have Any Weight to Reduce?

To lose weight, the Optimum Weight 5 and 1 plan is intended. We suggest the Optimum Health 3and 3 plan if you don't have weight to lose but want to make your eating habits better. This plan aims to assist you in maintaining a good weight in a refreshing manner and nutritionally balanced.

With the Lean and Green Program, What Ingredients and Good Fats Will an Individual Have?

To include zest and flavor in your meals, make sure they relate to the total carbohydrate intake. We suggest that the people go through the food labels for knowing about carbohydrates and information on condiment portions controlling for maximum results for optimum outcome.

A serving of condiments must contain not over than 1g per serving of carbohydrate. Individuals may take up to 3 condiment portions of each lean and green meal each day. Recommendations on Good Fat: Polyunsaturated and Monounsaturated fats such as avocado, olive oil, seeds and nuts, and olives are more effective for an individual's health than saturated fats. Among those two types, we recommend selecting most of your good fat servings. There must be no more than 5g of carbs and 5g of fats for a healthy fat meal. Based on the lean protein options, you can have 0 to 2 portions of good fats for each Lean and Green meal.

How Many Services Are Offered by Lean and Green?

Several programs to encourage Lean and Green provide optimal well-being. We help you improve your weight and improve your vitality, health, and focus while promoting healthy behaviors. Lean and Green services include:

- Optimal Weight Plan 5 and 1
- Optimal Weight Plan 4 and 2 and 1

- Optimal Weight Plan 5 and 2 and 2
- Optimum Health Plan 3 and 3
- Lean and Green for Pregnant Mothers
- Lean and Green for patients having diabetes
- Lean and Green for people (65 years and older)
- Lean and Green for boys (teenagers between 13 to 18)
- Lean and Green for girls (teenagers between 13 to 18)

Our most common weight loss program is the Ideal Weight 5 and 1 plan. Still, we also provide other plans to meet individuals' needs and preferences. To know all about these choices, we suggest you speak with the Lean and Green Mentor and then consult your health professional to decide which plan is right for you.

To Supplement Individuals' Programs, What Other Items Does Lean and Green Give?

Lean and Green provides a range of items to boost the regimen, including Lean and Green snacks, home meal flavors, Medifast Omega supplements for diet, and flavor infusers.

How Much Is It Going to Cost?

You'll buy the food upon selecting your schedule. Prices differ and rely on what and how many you're purchasing. The Optimal Critical Package comes along with 119 food servings (including shakes, sides, soup, bars, and snacks) for $414.60, combined with its optimal plan Weight 5 and 1. The 3 and 3 Plan's Ideal Wellness Package contains 130 food portions of related products for $333.

Will A Diet Work for Lean and Green?

The estimated weight reduction on the Optimum Weight 5 and 1 Plan is 12 pounds in around 12 weeks, as per the company.

On Lean and Green, How Much an Individual Can Eat?

According to the plan, Lean and Green recommends eating six to seven times a day (almost every 2 to 3 hours). The three available plans are:

- Plan 5 and 1: Eat 5 Lean and Green fuel items and 1 "Lean and Green" meal a day.
- Plan 4 and 2 and 1: Eat 4 Lean and Green fueling items, 2 "Lean and Green" meals, and one snack a day.
- Plan 3 and 3: Eat 3 Lean and Green Fuelings and 3 "Lean and Green" meals every day.

Is the Lean and Green Diet the Same as The Medifast?

A little bit. Medifast Inc. is Lean and Green's parent company. You can recall the Medifast service in the '80s and '90s, which had doctors recommending meals to the customers, is now owned and run. Lean and Green uses different foods with similar macronutrient intake profile, but customers should sign up electronically for the program themselves.

Do the Dietitians Recommend Lean and Green ?

Although being on Lean and Green will help you lose weight quickly, many dietitians are not big fans. Following the diet states that it cannot be a long-term option, while the diet may kick start weight loss. The supplement does not succeed in the long term, and you continue to focus on pre-packaged prepared meals and snacks. Instead, try to find a solution that suits your needs better so that you might get the outcomes you want.

What Salad Dressings Are Approved for The Lean and Green Diet?

The Lean and Green diet plan has a comprehensive range of famous brands such as Wishbone, Annie's Naturals, Newman's Own, Hidden Valley, Kraft, and Ken's. But, makes sure that your dressing amounts should not exceed two tablespoons in a single meal.

On the Lean and Green Diet, What Amount of Proteins Can You Get?

A "Lean and Green" meal contains 5 to 7 ounces of lean protein, and you'll still get a lot more protein from Fuelings. In general, on the Lean and Green diet, you can get 72 g of protein a day.

On the Lean and Green Diet, What Amount of Fats Can You Get?

You will have not more than 30 percent of the total calories (between 800 and 1,000) from the intake of fats. However, the Lean and Green diet's priority is healthy fats.

Hopefully, all your questions are answered within this final guide. Indeed, this is not the ending, but your starting point to achieve all your goals in your Lean and Green journey! Happy, healthy eating!